Loosen the Reins

A Recovery Journey to
Peace, Love, and Freedom

Jessie Miller

MY EPIC WRITING

Back cover photo provided by EPIC Outreach.

This book would not have been possible without the invaluable guidance and expertise of Beth Mansbridge and Nancy Quatrano, whose support in editing and publishing has been instrumental. I am deeply grateful for their contributions.

Published 2024 by My EPIC Writing, Jacksonville, Florida.

Printed in the United States of America.

I dedicate this book to *you*.

I hope you picked it up looking for inspiration to live on purpose for the highest good of yourself, others, and the planet.

To my husband, Jack—the kindest, most supportive soul on earth—thank you for your patience and unconditional love while you often play a secondary role to the other passions in my life.

And to the animals, who have been my true healers and teachers—those who have gone before, are here now, and those in the future—forever in my heart, they will remain as my greatest inspirations.

A special tribute goes to Wrigley the dog. I had you the longest time, and you walked with me on my journey of sobriety and abstinence from bulimia.

To Winnie, my little southern heart dog, I love you to the moon and back, and forevermore.

Of course, Taz and Kody—the horses who started it all—and to Oliver, Patches, Jimmy, and Moonpie, who taught me about pigs and made me want to save them all.

"Whether or not you know it, you're the infinite potential of love, peace, and joy."

—*Amit Ray*

Contents

Letter to My Readers

Dear Friend,

Yes, you, holding this book. If you picked up this book, I consider you a friend. We have something in common. I consider you a kindred spirit or a friend I have or haven't yet met.

My name is Jessie, and I'm pleased you're joining me on this journey of exploration. I am excited to tell you my story. Please know everything I spill out over these pages is being shared with the best intentions to inspire and help you see we are more alike than different. I mean no harm to anyone, and if I can help one person, I've done my part.

Wherever you are in life, I want you to know *you matter*!

I hope you are in a good place and are ready to be inspired. You are a magical being, you are beautiful, and you are loved!

Thank you for showing up today. Thank you for investing time in yourself. I imagine you are curled up with this book in your hands, ready to read, and ready to go with me. My wish is that you are relaxed in a cozy spot, drinking something yummy, and you have set aside some time to embrace and indulge in some reading fun for your heart and soul.

With you in mind, I have poured *my* heart and soul into this book. I also wrote it because I, too, needed to read and hear the words on these pages.

It's as if I am sitting with you and reading along as you sift through the words. My intent is for you to read as if we are sitting together and I am telling you my story.

And I promise this isn't a chance encounter; you are meant to be holding this book at this moment. I believe we are touched by things at the right time. No matter where you are in life, know this: it's perfect. Everything is exactly the way it is supposed to be.

This book is my invitation for you to connect with your soul, connect with the community around you, and find your voice so you can live the best, most authentic life you deserve.

Did you pick up this book because of the title? The reference to horses? I love horses, too. Maybe you liked the back cover text or perhaps someone suggested you might have a connection to the story.

However we came together, I will tell you I was originally inspired to tell my story to help others with an eating disorder (I will discuss that subject). As I collected content for the book through my experiences and awareness, I realized there was something deeper, something I wanted to highlight in hopes it shifts human beings into a new paradigm of thinking.

Every day we're alive, we can make a positive difference for ourselves and each other, for animals and the planet. We can make a difference by how we treat one another, how we use our platforms, like social media, to reach other people, and how—when we follow our passions—we have a more profound influence on the planet.

Over the past few years, I've gotten more fired up about life and love and the goodness this planet has to offer. It took me way too long to create this book and publish it due to the fact that I lived in a space of fear and worry and self-degradation. For days, weeks, months, and even years, this book called to my heart to be written. I ignored it.

Why?

I lacked the confidence to believe I had a story to tell. I didn't think I was worthy of writing, and who would want to read my story, anyway?

However, today I'm excited to tell you I enjoy an energy of love, joy, peace, hope, and freedom, and I want to share that energy with the world, with you!

Today I put one foot in front of the other and follow the guidance of my soul. I am inspired to not only tell my story, but to live an authentic life every moment forward. If those actions inspire even one person to choose a healthier, more joyful path for themselves, every doubt and struggle was worth it.

While I want this book to reach millions of people, I am okay if it inspires and changes the life of only one. That one person may be *you*. If that's the case, then writing this book accomplished its purpose. And you and I were meant to connect through the messages within these pages.

Whatever inspires you in life is perfect and magical and for your greater good.

As I continue to live, learn, and grow, I will gather new experiences and ideas. The new awareness will build on this book, so more books will come. We never arrive; we expand and rebuild and grow throughout our life.

You may be holding this book today, and a year or five years from now you'll pick it up and read it again and hear or see something in a new light, with a fresh perspective. That's because you have grown and evolved, and the ideas resonate in a different way. It happens to me with some books.

We build and refine from experiences. My invitation to you is to lean in and listen as the words resonate within your soul. Trust the process and, when inspired, take leaps of faith!

At the time of this book's printing, I live on a farm sanctuary (you'll learn more about it in the coming pages). The sanctuary is an inspiration: I had to create a space where rescued farm animals could later serve as education ambassadors to inspire kindness and compassion.

That creation required me to take a leap of faith.

When I envisioned the sanctuary and all it would do for the community and planet, I never dreamed I would be a fundraiser, a person who constantly asks others for money to support the cause. Being a fundraiser always had such an icky feeling to me. But to allow the sanctuary to exist, fundraising is something I had to learn to do every year, every month, sometimes weekly, sometimes daily.

I am constantly searching for creative ways to connect people to the mission, to support the work. And while at first it was not the vision I had originally seen, today it is a labor of love. I have fallen in love with fundraising.

I cannot see myself doing anything else—that is, except writing. I do love to write.

This book is another way I will be able to generate funding support for the sanctuary and the mission. A portion of the sales will go directly to the animals and education outreach, so your purchase and reading of this book will make a difference for others. Thank you!

Leaps of faith happen, and we never know where they will take us. All we must do is trust the process. My wish for you is that you are guided to your own calling; may this book lead you one step closer to your path.

It is with the greatest gratitude I thank you for taking the time to follow along with me on this journey. Let's begin!

Jessie

Beginnings

It took me four years to write this book! I hemmed and hawed for years. I didn't think I had a story worth telling. But every single time I asked the universe* what's next, I heard, loud and clear, "Write your dang book!"

In 2020 I buckled down to write and draft the first 40,000-word version. Over the next year it sat on the shelf collecting dust. I heard the nudging to write the book and get it done, but I always found something else to do.

In 2021 the calling to write got stronger, and I had several encounters during the summer which lit the fire under my butt to take action.

While walking on the beach with my sister and my husband, I saw a gal who was emaciated.

Skin and bones.

She was with her friend, and I'm sure she had no clue how skinny she was.

I knew.

I could feel her pain. I wanted to go hug her and tell her she mattered. I wanted to tell her she was gorgeous, no matter what she thought.

But I knew until someone is ready to face the music and make up their mind to get better, they never will. For years people told me I was beautiful, and while I heard the words, I couldn't grasp that truth. What I saw staring back in the mirror was flaw after flaw after flaw. My arms were too jiggly, my face too puffy, and my stomach had a "pouch" with rolls.

I was not happy with my body—ever.

A few weeks later, I was sitting on the beach soaking up some solitude, when I witnessed two teenage girls hanging out. As I watched them, I reminisced about my early years of carefree living.

One girl was more confident than the other. The other wouldn't take her shirt off. She wanted to; she kept pulling it up as if she was going to, but she was insecure, looking around to see who might spot her in her bathing suit.

By society's standards, the girls were both in great shape: not fat, not too skinny. They were young and vibrant and full of life.

But the one girl with the shirt ....

I could see and sense her insecurity and saw myself in her: afraid of who might see her on the large expanse of beach with people far and wide.

No one was watching them but me, and no one cared. That's the reality of the disease of perception. We think everyone is watching us and cares about us or how we look. Most people do not. We're our own worst critic.

And lastly, there were a few conversations I had with a dear friend who has a child in middle school.

Her daughter is already experiencing insecurities about her body image and comparing herself to her friends. My own addiction began in high school. If I could go back in time and tell younger Jessie not to waste so much time and energy on her body and insecurities—there is so much more to life—I would in a heartbeat!

Those three incidents in 2021 made me get down to writing. Living with an eating disorder disease for so long, and finally breaking free of it, made me want to inspire others to break free from the same crippling disorders.

Honestly, I want people to be free of *whatever* is crippling them.

What has *you* by your throat, suffocating you—something you can't see a way out of?

For me it was: body dysmorphia, a desire to please others, my ego, lack of self-confidence, and a lack of love for myself. I saw myself in the three scenarios I just related, and the pain was nearly unbearable. I was able to get out from under the body image stuff that had me in a vise grip, and I feel like it's a miracle.

Truthfully, though, anyone can break free. We all have access to freedom; it lies within.

As I began to understand emotional freedom, I developed a deep desire to tell my story to help others find freedom for themselves.

When I had doubts about recounting my story, I kept hearing a message from within. God said: *You do have something to share. You overcame bulimia, and hundreds of thousands of people are suffering with an eating disorder, even people you probably know. You overcame the bingeing and purging of every day of your life for twenty plus years. Tell your story to help someone else.*

Why do we honor people for "losing weight"? Why can't we be content with people of all sizes and shapes? We live in a diverse world. So the pressure to be a certain size or shape is bogus. God loves me all the way around, and he loves every one of us, not our size or shape, but for who we are, created in the likeness and image of our Creator.

I'm not an anomaly; many men and women face this disease right now. Eating disorders plague so many people. What I am is a voice that won't stay silent anymore.

Let's talk about how society puts such pressure and parameters on "what we should look like."

I was insecure and came out of the womb afraid of my own shadow, always standing behind my mother. I did things alone, not with friends, for fear of being ridiculed. I was the last person picked for kickball and any other sports activity. I was insecure as a child from the beginning, but animals, alcohol, and food made me feel validated and alive.

I can't get someone to be sober or keep them sober. I can't make someone abstain from an eating disorder. I only disclose my story in the hopes my experience inspires someone to choose a better path for themselves, to live a more healthy and abundant life.

I did.

I loosened the reins!

Today I've learned to dance with my body. Diets don't work for me—they are too limiting. I do better by asking my soul what it needs and how might I best serve it today. I go within and ask my body, connect to the cells, muscles, organs, and comingle with their energy. I assure my body I love it—by deeply connecting to my body and soul and saying thank you, I love you, and I'm here for you.

It's what I ultimately did to move beyond the blockage and reach freedom.

I don't have a wall covered with educational degrees. I don't have a blueprint of how I overcame the addiction of bingeing and purging, so I dragged my feet in writing this book. Why would people want to read my book?

What I've come to believe is we all need the encouragement and inspiration we gain from hearing other stories so we can say "me too." We need to come out with our stories so other people who feel ashamed or alone can believe they can do it too. So while I will pass along some ways of how I became and still stay abstinent, they are not the only ways to heal from addiction. If you find something to help nudge you in overcoming an addiction, then please use it. If something inspires you, please implement it into your own life. We each have a path and no one's path looks, feels, or is the same.

I started by looking within.

I often visit the ocean and look out at the water. Beneath the surface is a vast sea of life. You and I cannot see below the surface from the vantage point of walking on the beach, but we know lots of fish, sharks, plants, turtles, and so on live in the ocean, out of sight. An abundance of life thrives in that large body of water.

The same thing is going on inside of us. Our hearts pump endless amounts of blood. Our lives are full. Inside us is abundance—cells, organs, muscle and nerve systems. It's vast and full of love and light. Our insides are no different than a millionaire's insides and therefore our insides mirror that of a millionaire. We are an attractor to the outside of what's on the inside.

You believe you are a millionaire on the inside; therefore you *must* be a millionaire on the outside.

These many awakenings finally led me to take the time to complete this book.

In 2022, after a deep edit of the memoir, I again left the book sitting on my nightstand, afraid to read the critique and edits from the editor I had paid to help me.

I was afraid I was going to be told the book was a failure and I didn't have any right to write this memoir. It sat for several months until I learned of the passing of a friend of a friend who was younger than me.

She died of anorexia.

She was a beautiful soul inside and out. I sat in disbelief, hearing the news, and asked, "Why? How does this happen?"

Of course I thought of my book manuscript sitting and collecting dust. I thought, *I can't help anyone if I don't tell my story.*

So I picked up pen and paper and began to write. And, despite the rigid inner critique of my self-image, I set out not only to publish this book at long last, but to find peace with my own self-worth and love.

I feel more grounded today than at any other time in my life. I know good things are happening for me. And they can happen for you too!

I know my life is worthy and my experiences have value. I know now that I live a beautiful, abundant, and loving life of love, joy, peace, ease, and abundance—so much abundance.

It's through self-love and understanding, and finding joy, peace, and freedom in life that I share this book with you.

(*Author's note: When I mention God, the universe, and prayer, I invite you to look past whatever your beliefs might be regarding spirituality. We each have our own understanding of a higher power; I'm not trying to change your beliefs. My goal is to invite you to follow along with me and my awakening so you might find something here to help you in your own healing and consequent freedom.)

How It All Started

In the Alcoholics Anonymous (AA) program, which I'll talk more about later, I learned to tell my story of sobriety with a beginning, a middle, and an end.

What was it like before, how did it change, and what's it like today?

So I'm going to use the same format, mostly.

Let's start at the beginning.

Growing up in a middle-class household seemed ordinary; it was all I knew. I had a mom and a dad who were married and I was the middle child between two sisters. Mom stayed home to take care of us girls, and Dad worked two jobs. He was rarely around, always traveling or working.

We lived with food on the table every night and some hand-me-down clothes. I had everything I desired: a dog, a Barbie doll, a Cabbage Patch Kid doll, a Pound Puppy, and did I mention a real-life family pet dog? Yes, I would say our life in that small New Jersey town was great.

We often visited the boardwalk at Seaside Heights, long before it became popular as the *Jersey Shore* reality television series. The little blue house where I spent my early childhood years was big to me, but visiting it now, as an adult, it's like a postage stamp. Still, it was ours and we loved it.

Our backyard was fenced for our dog to run and play in, and we had a swing set in the backyard, built by my dad and my

1

grandfather. I even had a little garden on the side of the house where I grew marigolds.

I loved to run across the street to the little red house, where my best friend Sarah lived.

Woodland Drive was full of kids growing up together, playing, laughing, and learning in the wooded lot the homes strategically circled. We kids zoomed around the blocks, up and down the roads on our bikes, always paying attention to the street lights, an indication when they came on it was time to head home for dinner, unless we heard my mom ring the bell.

The neighborhood was small enough that the little handheld bell could be heard several streets away. And the sound of the bell meant you had better get home quick.

It was a safe neighborhood.

It was cozy inside our tiny home. Mom and Dad were always rearranging rooms and walls made of dressers and cardboard barriers to create new spaces.

Three girls, two parents, and a dog in a two-bedroom, one-bathroom home. It was tight, yet we managed as a family.

My home in that neighborhood is where I cultivated my love for animals.

My Love for Animals Began Early

It is as if I came out of the womb an animal lover. From my earliest memories I recall having a gift with animals. I was instantly and always drawn to animals of any kind. When I played with my friends I always played with stuffed animals. I was not a big baby doll fan. I didn't want to play house and have a husband, the house, and the kids.

I wanted the animals, including dogs, cats, horses, and bunnies.

My first encounter with kittens was at the Wawa on Drum Point Road, where I visited with my grandmother. It wasn't the Wawa convenience stores and gas stations most are familiar with today. Grandma's Wawa in the early 1980s was more like your local town convenience store with a fruit and vegetable stand. Kittens were always running in, around, and under the pallet displays of food. I caught and cuddled those hissy, spitting things, and my grandma cooed over them, calling them "cunning."

On the same road was Osbornville Elementary School. I rode the bus to and from school, along the road where I had the encounter with a German shepherd that would begin to pave the path for my future. I was barely ten years old when one day, on the ride home from school, I witnessed a beautiful rust-and-black-colored German shepherd dog lying motionless in the street.

The bus driver had stopped for traffic after seeing the dog get hit by a car.

I stared out the window at the lifeless body.

As I looked down from my seat on the big yellow bus, I thought, *Where is its owner? Why is no one doing anything? Why doesn't anyone care?*

He lay there helpless and homeless on the black pavement—dead.

At that moment I knew deep down inside there was a greater calling on my life. The seed for working with and advocating for animals got planted and began to grow. I knew I was going to do something that would save, protect, and make a difference for all things.

Thirty-two years later, I started a farm sanctuary where I began to care for a homeless horse named Kody—who would change the course of my life!

But first, in my early years I set out to learn as much as I could about animals of all kinds. I began to save every newspaper article which talked about animals: from stories about captive animals in zoos, to heartwarming stories about man's best friend, or pictures of featured pets looking for homes at the local animal shelter. My grandmother clipped articles and pictures and saved them for me, and my dad photocopied library books I fell in love with.

I kept the images and information to review and read and study. I became obsessed with learning anything and everything I could about animals.

Dad's job took us overseas to live in a small town called Worms, a city in Germany. While we were fortunate to see many cool things, like Big Ben, the Autobahn, and the fall of the Berlin Wall, it always felt like we were on the move and constantly making new friends. While living overseas I didn't have a dog for a while, but my parents let me have my first personal pet, a red-eared slider.

I was in middle school and still absorbing everything I could about animals. I didn't understand the concept of pet stores and keeping animals in captivity. We bought the little turtle from a German pet store, and I loved it like it was my baby. I am not even sure if it was a girl or a boy, but to me the green-shelled cutie was a girl. I named her Tucy (pronounced Too-sea). I spent time with Tucy like you would a dog or a cat, letting her have time to crawl in our backyard grass or in my room. I even wrote a children's story about Tucy and her adventures.

Tucy was my door to creativity and learning to care for a pet. When Dad got transferred back to the United States and we had to find a place for my turtle friend to go, it was my first encounter with saying goodbye to a beloved pet.

We did a lot of sightseeing travel while living in Europe and during our travels we stayed in many different hotels. One hotel in Holland had a huge, indoor, well-cared-for turtle pond. I distinctly remember being fascinated by the happy turtles which looked like my Tucy.

Our family planned a release trip to that hotel where I was able to secretly set Tucy free into the oasis with the other sliders. Looking back, I know Tucy may not have survived, but in my preteen knowledge and awareness at the time, it was the best thing I could do for my beloved turtle friend.

Our family transferred to Cape Cod, Massachusetts, where I began my high school years. When I was at age fifteen, my eating disorder started and alcohol entered the scene.

But before I tell you about that, let me tell you about my friend Sarah.

A Best Friend Named Sarah

Two of Hearts, Two Hearts That Beat as One

She lived across the street in the "little red house." As kids growing up together, we played daily. She was known as "Big Sarah" in the neighborhood; she was tall and older than "Little Sara." She was on the cheerleading squad, she was beautiful, and she cared deeply for her younger siblings.

Sarah was my best friend. We were inseparable as kids, playing every chance we had, hanging out at my house or hers.

> We bought one of those gold chain necklaces with the charm that split down the middle and read "Best Friends;" she kept one half and I had the other. We laughed and played and did everything together.

One of my fondest memories was when we did a skit to the song "Two of Hearts" by Stacy Q. Who remembers Stacy Q? She is an American pop singer from the 1980s.

We recited and practiced the skit for a long time before performing it in her backyard for our families. It was the going-away skit, our final time together before my family and I moved away when we got transferred by my dad's job.

We moved from New Jersey to Texas and then to Germany.

The song, the skit, the fun in her backyard is the lasting memory I have of her. Those lyrics will forever ring in my head: "Two of hearts, two hearts that beat as one." We were two hearts that beat as one, a friendship like no other.

Her friendship left an impression on my soul. It was a once-in-a-lifetime friendship. A rare, unique, cherished, instant connection. I was eleven years old going on twelve. Not even a teenager, but her friendship was imprinted on my soul as we grew during those early years of our lives.

She was my best friend.

While living thousands of miles away in Germany in the late 1980s, our family received a message from my grandmother. The message came through a telegraph because then, social media and cell phones did not exist.

Tragically, Sarah was killed in a car accident. At the time I received that earth-shattering news, I was twelve years old. We were living in civilian housing and I had an upstairs bedroom. I isolated myself and didn't want to talk to anyone. In looking back, I discovered that was when my emotional distortion began.

My grief was constant. I couldn't return home to the States to say goodbye to my friend. I had to grieve while already feeling displaced in a foreign country and ripped away from the normalcy of the things we knew and loved while growing up. I was never able to say goodbye to her in person and it left a big hole in my soul.

School authorities and my parents arranged for me to speak to a grief counselor in school. It felt forced and inauthentic, like it was a routine thing to do when a child experienced loss. Their parents sent them off to counseling. They'd be fine.

I didn't want to talk about anything, yet there I was, sitting in a room with a stranger to talk about my feelings. I didn't get the chance to process and feel my feelings. I was forced to move them along, share them with a stranger—yuck—and pretend I was getting better.

I went through the motion of emotions I was expected to show. It was the thing to do to make my parents happy. But what I wanted was to have my friend back and I wanted to go say goodbye to her in person. I wanted to hug her again, laugh with her, run across the street when her mom's station wagon pulled into the driveway, and ask my friend to make leaf houses in the front yard. I wanted us to shake our fannies to the beat of "Two of Hearts" and pretend we were Suzie Q.

The pure authentic love of that childhood friendship, a connection of innocence, of having a friend I grew up with and had plans to grow through life with, was stolen from me.

Not getting to say goodbye to my "other half" left me helpless and sad.

Truly sad.

At some point, my mom told me my grandmother had attended the funeral and took carnations on behalf of my sisters and me. She placed those carnations in the casket.

While today I understand the reasons why I was not able to leave Germany to fly home to say goodbye to my friend, at the time I began the practice of making up stories about relationships.

I made up a story so I would not care too much. Later in life, when painful things happened, the fables allowed me to brush events and pain off like they weren't important. I created a story about not getting close to people because of my intense fear of losing a person I cared deeply for. Getting close to someone was too painful a risk, so I distanced myself from others.

Looking back through my recovery, I could see how, as I ventured into adulthood, that method of operating showed up in my subconscious actions.

I never attended funerals. I found excuses not to go; after all, final goodbyes don't matter. Today I still work hard to muster the courage to go to a funeral or "celebration of life," often making excuses to avoid the feelings of loss, no matter how close I am to someone.

An emptiness settled within me. I wanted closure and didn't get it. I remember feeling a deep sadness, and everyone around me wanted to fix it. All I wanted was to have my friend back or at least have the chance to go say goodbye.

During that time, a feeling of abandonment came my way, and food became my solace. Building new friendships was hard. I was afraid everyone was going to leave me, and the fear carried all the way into adulthood. Food never disappointed me. It was always there and it was always comforting. The experiences in our childhood years often create subconscious responses we carry with us as we go through life. Most of the time, we don't even recognize what we're doing is a response to the initial childhood experience.

As an adult, I found myself brushing things off, not making a big deal about them. I had a hard time trusting anyone or anything, subconsciously afraid I'd be abandoned. Safer not to get too close than losing someone or something I've grown to love.

But some things have healed over time. Not accidentally, of course.

When we finally do some deep-healing, soul-searching work, we uncover the stories we've created that dictate how we live our life. And realize how we respond to and process our experiences. Once we unpack those stories and begin to unravel them, we can create new paths for living.

Through a program of recovery and the creation of an education farm sanctuary, I have learned new ways to trust and live.

Being on the farm and spending time with the horses, especially the one who bit me, has given me the space to relive those times with my best friend. I allow for healing and peace with all that is, was, and is to come. I have found when I slow down and work with big, amazing creatures like horses, they have more to teach me than I can teach them. I'm learning that my slower, understanding approach is causing me to be mindful of the horses, which in turn allows me the space to exhale those years of bottling things up and holding on to hurt feelings and negative emotions.

I share the story of Sarah because these kinds of experiences—whether they happen when we are a child or later in life—can sometimes change how we respond and proceed with life, altering our lives forever.

It takes time, healing, the rewiring of our thoughts, feelings, and actions to carve a new response and create the new life we desire to live.

The Influence of Ego

We lived on Cape Cod, where I attended high school. My love for animals continued to grow.

We settled in a town called Centerville, which happened to be home to one of the animal shelters of the Massachusetts Society for the Prevention of Cruelty to Animals (MSPCA). It didn't take me long to begin visiting and volunteering, spending as much free time at the shelter as possible.

I loved it.

After school, the school bus would drop me off on Falmouth Road / Rte. 28. I volunteered for the afternoon and sometimes I got picked up by my mom or was given a ride home by one of the employees. When there was no ride available, I walked home.

Being able to walk dogs, feed and clean up after the cats, and help in any way the staff would let me, invigorated my soul. Over the years I saw the shelter through staff changes and reorganization, and I learned a great deal about animal care and animal sheltering. Some of it was hard truths about pet overpopulation and the reality of making daily decisions of life and death. I also got to learn about veterinary care, incinerators, and doing wildlife rescue calls for raccoons, skunks, and wild birds.

In 1995, after I graduated from high school, the MSPCA hired me as one of their full-time staff.

I was elated.

It was the first step to the beginning of my animal welfare career. It was also when I learned about the ego.

I've learned our ego is the thing behind everything we do. The ego can and will drive our decisions, reactions, and actions almost every time. So, what is ego?

Ego represents every human's sense of self-identity and self-importance. It includes our awareness of ourselves and the perceptions of ourselves as different from others.

When I feel the overpowering need to get my point across, it's my ego driving me. When I feel I must prove myself, that's my ego, too. Competition with one another is driven by ego. Seeking to be the top dog or get all the attention, hog the spotlight—all ego.

As an avid and lifelong animal advocate, I've witnessed ego get in the way of saving lives. The actual act of lifesaving can be more about people's personal agendas than the welfare of the animals they claim to care about. I've been guilty of this too, on occasion, since the ego has a subtle way of creeping into everything we do if we aren't paying attention. I've learned good management of our ego is important for personal growth and healthy relationships, as well as our overall well-being. But if we aren't aware of our egos, we can do a lot of damage, some of it irreparable.

A wise leader once said, "The ego kills more animals," and I knew exactly what she meant.

Not Aligning to the Popular Vote

In 1996, a time when animal shelters were making decisions daily on animals' lives, I was working for the MSPCA. Millions of dogs and cats were dying in shelters. The pet overpopulation was at an all-time high and decisions were being made if an animal lived or died based on their health, temperament, if there was space in the shelter, how long an animal had been at the shelter, and even the color of the animal.

The thinking was: A shelter full of black-and-white cats or dogs wouldn't offer enough variety to those looking to adopt a new pet. The sad truth is a variety of colors, shapes, sizes, and ages of animals helps to increase adoptions. This fact plays a part in which animals get to live and be on the adoption floor, even today. Yes, the same situations still occur in many animal shelters across the globe/nation even though the number of animals being euthanized in shelters today has significantly decreased. We've made some progress in rehoming and fostering animals, but there's still a lot of work to do.

This story I'm about to tell you is from my early days as an animal shelter worker.

As I plunged into the beginning of my animal welfare career, it was when this crazy selection process of who lives and who dies was taking place. It was a time when the pit bull dog breed was horribly misunderstood.

The pit bull breed is still misunderstood, but back then it was even worse. Many people and society in general associated this breed of dog with dogfighting and being a menace to society. The breed had a sordid reputation, which created fear in people. The unwanted dogs landed in shelters as strays or were surrendered by owners simply because of the breed.

Condo and homeowner groups banned them and forced pet owners to surrender them, and insurance companies refused to insure a family or home if they owned one. The scenario was not good for this terrier.

Misconceptions and misinformation about the breed led animal shelters to make decisions about the dogs' lives which were irrational and, unfortunately, biased and unfair to the dog.

For example, if a mom pit bull dog came in with marks on her body which "looked like dogfighting marks," and she had an unknown history as a result of being picked up with puppies as a stray, the decision was often made instantly to euthanize, or kill, those puppies rather than place them up for adoption and risk having a "vicious" dog in the community.

It was thought that the urge to "fight to the death" was bred into a dog and if one was picked up and a fight history was suspected, it was a death sentence for the dog. Therefore, unless you could be 100 percent certain an adult mom dog didn't come from a fighting line or dogfighting ring, the shelter wouldn't take the risk of adoption for fear that dog might someday maul a human; after all, they were a "fighter."

The mom and puppies scenario became a reality for me in 1996, when a female pit bull came into the shelter with the cutest puppies who were only six weeks old. She was a dark chocolate brown with black and blonde brindle colors in her short-haired coat. Her puppies were a mix of her colors, and some were black-and-white. The mom dog had scar-type marks on her legs, nose, and chest area, and since she had an unknown history, it led the staff to believe she had been part of a dogfighting ring—based on her appearance and nothing else.

There was no proof the mom dog had been in a dogfighting ring; she exhibited no signs of aggression toward people. She sat tied in the intake holding area of the shelter. She was sweet and docile when you approached her to say hello. And, the truth is, often the breed doesn't show aggression to humans. Many don't want to fight with other dogs either, but it's the situation they're placed in which forces them to act the way they do. The human handlers use various cruel tools to provoke and instigate them to fight with others.

The mom dog's behavior didn't indicate she was a fighter. That categorization was something made up by stereotypical hype at the time. But because of the myths associated with the breed, it was automatically assumed her tiny puppies were "bred to be fighters." The decision was made to end their lives. It was not worth the risk to the public to adopt those dogs out as pets and risk their growing up to be "biters."

I'd met the mother dog and puppies when they first came into the shelter, but I was not at the shelter or part of the decision to end their lives the day it was made. When I came in and learned the outcome, I was furious.

I was only nineteen or twenty years of age, and I didn't handle my feelings or emotions well. I was right, I was angry, and I was outraged. I remember being terribly upset—which I now recognize as my ego—and I chose to serve my ego by storming out of the shelter in a rage of crying and angry emotion. I couldn't control the outcome, no matter how much I pleaded and bartered for those puppies' lives. I knew deep down the decision and the reasons for the decision were not right, but I didn't have a platform to stand on, nor the guts and courage to constructively stand up and prevent it.

I was young, inexperienced, and a meek person. I was loud and aggressive and fierce on the inside, but I didn't know how to express myself in an effective manner, so I chose to serve my ego. I felt like I didn't have a voice and my input didn't matter. My ego insisted I wasn't able to control the situation; therefore, all I could do was throw a mini temper tantrum and storm out like a two-year-old who was told they couldn't have dessert.

The ego is part of our human makeup. It's something human beings can't opt out of. And it's up to each of us to choose how we let ego affect our life.

Do we serve our ego or do we let our ego serve us? Tricky, I know. Letting my ego serve me is not about proving myself, but about being transparent and showing up, acknowledging the truth about things, and allowing energy to move things forward rather than making everything be about me.

Ending the lives of those dogs was a tragic decision, and today, looking back, I can see the rationale behind it. It was made based on what people understood at the time. When we know better, we do better. But the way I handled the situation demonstrates how I reacted face-to-face with my ego and my insecurities in an adult situation.

If I could go back and change how I responded, I would have asked them to take a leap, to try something new, and approach the situation from a different perspective.

I would have been a louder voice for those innocent animals. The incident is so engraved into my memory, it has made me evaluate, as I grow, how I let ego serve or not serve me. It has made me open my mind to see things differently and not to rely solely on what someone else says. I step back today and look at things thoroughly before I make an important decision.

My ego can show up as it did in this situation, masked as a spoiled child. I see it in others too, and when you spot it, you got it. When I recognize it in others, I always know to check *myself*. Ego isn't always bad; it can either drive ambition and success, or lead to arrogance and insecurity. What's important is having the ability to recognize when ego is either serving us or we're serving it.

The story is applicable to any situation. It's a story I remember and reflect on, wishing I'd had the voice I have today. I wish I'd known then how to speak up for those dogs.

Read the story and put it in context for a relatable subject you connect with in your life. Maybe you're a social worker helping kids and families, maybe you're a researcher, or you work for the airline industry—whatever arena you're in, I'm sure you can relate to the premise of this story. It's about ego, about losing your voice, and maybe going with the popular vote.

It took me a long time to overcome my ego.

My Ego Makes Me Feel Like a Fraud!

Fast-forward twenty plus years and I'm still learning and understanding this ego thing. Right now, as I type this book, I'm conscious of serving my ego again, but with a lot less judgment.

Writing this book has put me in the face of my ego like few other tasks or events have. Initially, when writing this book, I felt like a fraud. I had no idea where to begin. My ideas were all over the place. Asking for help is something I've always done, but writing is so personal and asking for help with editing was not something I thought to do.

My brain is like a scrambled egg: fried, fluffy, and full of salt and pepper. Ha! My brain never shuts up: it's like a dash of this and a dash of that, look over here, look over there. The crazy scrambled-ness can usually be pointed at my ego; I try to do more, more, more, in a hurried way, to prove my worth by the things I accomplish. Ultimately it took so long to write this book because my ego kept getting in the way. I wanted to tell my story ... but didn't want to reveal the muck and mire for fear you would judge me and not like me. My ego wants everyone to like me. I thought you would judge my writing, and my ego couldn't bear the thought you might say I could have or should have done better in the writing of this memoir.

Yup, it's disturbing how our minds make up so many stories and crazy lies. And the insecurities? That's ego. My ego overcompensated to make up for my unworthy, low self-esteem feelings.

While I say I felt like a fraud to be writing this book and revealing deep introspections, I think about where that idea comes from: my ego. It's a place of wanting to be perfect before I do anything or create anything. I want to have everything lined up seamlessly and until it is, I'm not going to move on it.

I felt like a fraud. This book is about overcoming addiction and low self-esteem, which are both rooted in the ego. This book is about overcoming an eating disorder that had me by the throat for twenty-five plus years of my life. It's about a "pouch"—which is how I view my belly. Today I still loathe the pouch at times, but we're slowly becoming friends. That's also part of what I want you to understand. Acceptance and honest love take time and the work is never done. It's okay.

I felt like a fraud; I still need to work at loving myself completely, on a daily basis. I must constantly look in the mirror and reassure myself I'm perfectly perfect. I'm not the flaws; instead, I celebrate the things that are gorgeous and exciting!

As a wise person once told me, if we waited for perfection, nothing would get done. Nothing would get written, nothing would get shared, art wouldn't get created, songs wouldn't get written, businesses wouldn't start.

I now accept I am not perfect; however, my ego wanted and still wants me to be perfect before I complete or send this book into the world—or before I complete or do anything. So I let my ego serve me by exposing my vulnerabilities of not being perfect, and work with it. This book sets me on the path of speaking to you, one-on-one, as a friend and an equal.

We are all perfect in our own unique ways. In Psalm 139, David writes to God and says, "I am fearfully and wonderfully made." Scholars feel the passage points out that we are each created with care and great attention to each detail, by our Creator. We are perfectly imperfect.

Each of us has something amiss, something which makes us unique and perfect in our own special ways. We started somewhere, being perfectly imperfect, to arrive where we are today. I may have more days ahead when I feel like a fraud, but the beautiful thing is I have the choice to acknowledge the thought and set it aside, or let it ruin my day. I either serve it or let it serve me.

As I move forward in life, I strive to always choose to allow those thoughts to serve me. I first acknowledge them and then pivot and choose a higher vibrational thought: I get to choose to move forward in a joyful, non-negative energy.

Because I say so, this book is serving as a platform I chose constructively, to be a voice for healing and truth while also inviting and inspiring healing and truth for others—for you—a power I didn't have when those puppies' lives were on the line.

Getting Sober

We all have a belly button birthday, which is the day we were born.

Every year since 2009, I celebrate a second birthday.

I'm a sober sister, and January 13, 2009, is my born-again day, when my life took a new path—in a positive direction. It's my sobriety date. Though drugs, alcohol, and an eating disorder are parts of my story, the eating disorder and alcohol drove me into sobriety. The eating disorder is what I'll talk about most; it's the underlying current that motivated me to write this book.

For full disclosure, the recounting of my experience is merely *my* experience, *my* opinions, and not those of any individual or group. I used a program of recovery and applied the principles and steps of a twelve-step program to get sober, which helped me to:

1. quit drinking and

2. quit being a raging bulimic.

Let's start with the addiction and where it began.

While I was volunteering at the animal shelter I was also coming into my own personality and learning things about myself through interactions with friends in and outside of school. I began drinking alcohol during my high school years. Discovering alcohol was a way not only to cope with life but to fit in with my peers.

The eating disorder also began then. It wasn't something I recognized as being out of control—yet today I can look back and see that while I was exhibiting addictive behaviors in many forms, what I was doing was stuffing feelings—not coping with life or emotions—and I had no idea how to live in a world without altering how I felt about myself or others.

Food, alcohol, and drugs were the substances I abused to cope with while growing up.

The three components were temporary alterations, so I did them over and over and over, seeking relief from life, whether due to work, family, relationships, money, or my inner emotional discord. The addiction was never-ending. Using food was how it started, but the alcohol quickly followed the food. Both things provided me immediate comfort. They were things I could control, which fueled the egomaniac within.

Alcohol and bulimia went hand in hand.

Deep within, I knew the eating disorder was abnormal; I mean, who binges and purges food? Humans must eat to survive. I knew I was abusing my body with food, but in my early years of drinking I didn't think alcohol was such a problem. I assumed everyone drank the way I did. Plus, I have many fond memories of drinking with friends on Cape Cod and outside of Boston, in Southwest Florida, and then in Northeast Florida where I would eventually get sober.

Many times, drinking was a social thing that eventually led to overindulging and isolation.

I grew up nurtured and loved. I got good grades in school; I even made the honor roll. When I was in high school, I started a small, lucrative side business while working part-time at the local animal hospital. I was a pet sitter for clients, and my parents trusted me, which allowed me to spend the night watching people's beloved animals.

I did overnights, driving myself to school for classes in the morning and letting the pets out at lunch and after school. It was a sweet gig for the early stages and beginning years of my eating disorder.

Pet sitting was a recipe for success to keep my bingeing and purging a secret. I was able to master the craft of bulimia behind closed doors. My pet sitting business gave me the opportunity to explode my eating disorder. I binged and purged to my heart's content in the privacy of those homes; it was perfect for fueling the thing that gave me validation and confidence in myself.

My ego was in full control. The bulimia quickly became a daily thing, and soon every time I ate and every time I thought of eating, it became a battle of the mind to control how I physically responded to food in my body.

Do I binge and purge, or not?

Many times, I couldn't wait to have a pet sitting job, especially the ones where I knew I would find good food options. I was free to binge and purge in ecstasy. Rather than my going out with friends, pet sitting gave me a valid excuse to stay in and indulge in yummy sugary foods. I stuffed my face until my stomach felt like it would explode, then followed by purging the food and calories away.

It was a vicious cycle: day after day, week after week.

Controlling how I looked—and banishing the dreaded belly pouch—made me feel like I was in control. I didn't know my ego was in charge. I didn't live life at a slow pace. Life was intense, always go-go-go. If I wasn't busy doing something, I considered myself unworthy and, by extension, my life was unworthy.

I lived under the misunderstanding that I had to be *doing* something to earn my value and worth, so I lived in a world of my own creation, where I was in control—creating chaos wherever I went, with whomever I encountered. I masked the emotions of my destruction through drinking, drugging, and eating in excess. Then I purged to control how I looked and felt. It was a crazy, crazy, wicked cycle and a miserable way to live.

Over the years I had bouts of abstinence from the eating disorder, but it never went away.

Note: The following paragraphs are detailed and graphic and could be a trigger for some still active in their addiction.

I became crafty in hiding the eating disorder and good at learning how to binge and purge quickly just about anywhere. I forced the vomiting until I felt all the food was up. I purged until bile came up from my stomach, the indicator I had gotten every bit of food out of my stomach.

Bile is wretched-tasting, and I know, after all those years of bingeing and purging, it ruined my teeth. Bile is acid-like and eats away at your teeth—from the backside.

When out to eat with friends or family, I knew the right stall to use in some restrooms, or it was a single powder room where I could purge in privacy. I got so good at my bulimic scheme I knew when to purge while standing in a stall, waiting for the precise timing of someone flushing a toilet so the regurgitation sounds were completely disguised by the flush.

Sometimes I would "go for a walk" to "clear my head and get some air," only to find a patch of woods where I could purge the food I'd just eaten at the family bar-b-que. I used grass and leaves to wipe my hands. Or I went to the basement to "do laundry" or hang out with the animals living there, only to purge my dinner in a plastic bag I could throw out with the kitchen trash.

Did people know?

I'm not sure, but I thought I had everyone fooled. I was a professional binger and purger. I spent a lot of money on food to soothe my soul. I piled up credit card debt and spent countless paychecks on junk food—cupcakes, chips, bagels, and drive-through greasy meals. It's insane the amount of money and food I wasted on that addiction.

I got good at knowing what foods would purge easily and what to drink to help those foods come up easier. I learned what foods did not come up easily and what not to drink. Water was not a good elixir, but milky substances or ones with bubbles were perfect. And I learned the liquid-to-food ratios which would cause food to regurgitate through my nostrils. It was always a nasty experience which often left me feeling like I didn't get all the food out of my stomach.

The goal was to empty my belly so I didn't feel "fat," much less *look* fat—a constant battle to look and feel thin and worthy of being liked and loved.

The drinking and bulimia helped me feel worthy, loved, and in control. If I wasn't bingeing and purging, I drowned my emotions of loneliness and insecurity in alcohol. It went on for years. I was into my early thirties before I finally got sober.

In 2008 I couldn't hold a job. I drank around the clock. It took every bit of energy to stay sober long enough to go to work and earn a paycheck. Though I lost a dream job I'd worked hard to attain, it was still not enough to keep me sober.

Looking back, I think the drinking had gotten out of hand a long time before 2008, but it was sure in my face when I lost my dream job. The alcohol addiction and eating disorder were identifiable contributing factors to that job loss. I often didn't show up to work in optimal condition and called in sick.

The bulimia was at full strength, happening every time I ate. It occurred with the drinking too, but I couldn't see past either one. Lord knows how many times I tried to control both, only to fail miserably. For someone so bent on controlling her life, there wasn't any aspect of my life under control.

I had to get a hold on one of them to be able to fix the other. After I lost my job, I had so much free time on my hands that the drinking got kicked up a notch. I began drinking every day, most of the day, until I couldn't take it anymore and neither could my roommates.

Since alcohol abuse was the biggest and most obvious hurdle, and I ultimately had to eat to survive, I was able to focus on addressing the alcohol. In 2009 I got into a treatment facility for alcoholism, which led to finally getting sober at the age of thirty-two.

I began to live a life of sobriety by following an Alcoholics Anonymous (AA) program.

Now, I would love to tell you as soon as I got sober, I stopped bingeing and purging, but I can't. I spent a long time in sobriety, working on rebuilding myself and learning a new way to function. I'm lucky and grateful I met many women in the AA program who dealt with eating disorders too, and I learned quickly I was not alone in having a dual disease—alcoholism *and* an eating disorder. But for some reason the eating disorder was not talked about much, and when it was mentioned, it was like it was being swept under the carpet.

Honestly, I didn't want to speak about it, either.

It was a guarded topic and since I was still actively doing it, I *really* didn't want to talk about it for fear of being judged. After all, the fear of being judged poorly—as insufficient and unworthy of love and respect—is what started my addictions. What a vicious circle.

Once you remove one addiction, if you're not careful, a new addiction can slip in and take its place. The food and bulimia were always there, but with the alcohol gone, food quickly became my vice and new best friend.

As I look back through my own filters, I don't think the bingeing and purging got worse, but it certainly didn't stop. I learned how to purge in the shower, or at least have the shower running to disguise the sound of throwing up. I did whatever I had to do to eat and not get caught getting rid of food. The creative, insidious ways I devised to control the food and how much I kept down for my body to use for nourishment—were absolutely amazing.

Looking at it now, I think it was probably borderline psychotic behavior. It took a lot of calculated thought to plan how and what I was going to eat, and when and where I would binge and purge. I was professional about it.

A popular definition of insanity is doing the same thing over and over and expecting different results. I would promise myself each month that things would be different and I would do better about the bingeing and purging, but I still kept doing it.

While in sobriety and working on overcoming the alcoholism, I was using the program of AA to stay sober, while also applying it to the eating disorder. I was talking with others and learning how they overcame their food obsessions. Things began to get better and I learned food could be my friend.

I did a lot of yo-yo dieting and became obsessed with running. I sometimes went for weeks and months without bingeing and purging episodes. I started to believe I had a handle on the food addiction, but I did relapse every so often.

Staying sober requires us to stay vigilant in our lifestyle, watching for our triggers and avoiding them if possible, being honest with ourselves always, and staying humble about our sobriety—which feels ultra fragile sometimes. Many years into my alcohol sobriety, I was so tuned in I started to recognize a pattern.

I relapsed most often with the eating disorder when I had my monthly feminine cycle, when my hormones shifted and things in my body changed. The weight gain and mood swings allowed me—and my ego—an excuse to use food to soothe those emotions and I'd be back in the clutches of bulimia.

It took a lot of work and practice to learn to sit through those feelings and let them go without having to feel like I had to get rid of every morsel of food I ate. It took ten years in sobriety and an encounter with a rescue horse named Kody before I eventually became abstinent from the eating disorder.

> Over time, I've taken a deep look within to loosen the reins on my soul so I could get to a place of surrender, in order to overcome the battle of bulimia addiction.

And like every recovery effort over every addiction, it's still a daily walk. That's where humility comes in. Ego and humility can't control us at the same time, so remembering I'm only one trigger or day or moment away from a drink or a binge and purge session is a mighty tool to staying away from those behaviors.

I'm vigilant and careful of what I eat and what time of the month it is, or when my body shifts and regulates, based on seasons and emotions. I know the trigger foods that will most likely take me out and I avoid them.

I talk about my addiction to food today in Alcoholics Anonymous meetings. It's a big part of my story, and I believe it needs to be disclosed to help others. It's the "why" for many people. While those meetings are focused on the abuse of alcohol, people have sometimes talked about other addictions. Most mention drugs, and not food or an eating disorder. I feel it's my responsibility to disclose more about this often-uncommunicated addiction—the more people talk about it, the less it's a taboo subject.

I'm not sure why people think the subject is off-limits or not important. *Many* people struggle with eating disorders, from bulimia to anorexia to overeating. I've been to a few Overeaters Anonymous meetings. The gatherings tend to stay in the problem more than in the solution, so it isn't my most powerful place. I don't attend them regularly. We must eat to survive and food is all around us. The world is driven by food: ads on television and marketing sensationalism surrounds sugary, salty, and fatty foods. Those kinds of foods taste yummy, but they start a phenomenon of craving which activates my need to purge. Those kinds of foods are my triggers.

I've lived with bulimia since I was fifteen years old—when I realized boys liked skinny girls. In elementary school I was picked on for being chubby and not having the best clothes. The bullying reinforced the lies my ego whispered to me over and over about being ugly and not worthy of good relationships with myself or others.

When I entered high school and realized the attention I got when I was thin, I made the connection again and thus the eating disorder began. At this point I also had an obsession for working out and eating minimally, focusing on what, how much, and when I ate. I obsessed over eating healthy foods and drinking lots of water. My relationship with food and my body self-image were off-balance. I had many obsessions back then, all in an effort to help me feel acceptable and to earn the admiration of others.

Those obsessions to gain the validation of others were based on my outer appearance, nothing more.

If we could go back and tell our younger selves something we know today but didn't back when we were young, what would we say?

I'd tell myself to stop trying so hard to be perfect. There's no such thing as perfection. Stop trying to be a certain way for someone else; we are enough, exactly the way we are. Stop comparing yourself to others. Be you and love yourself.

When I think about the energy we expend trying to please others and seeking what someone else has achieved, it's mind-boggling. The Bible has many warnings about wanting what others have. It is dangerous to our peace of mind and well-being.

To make matters much worse, especially for young people, social media is a breeding ground of judgments and comparisons and self-image nightmares. Wanting to look good to others, to fit in, or to impress others, we post our best selves out there to the world and hide the muck and mire. Look out, though, if the best self you posted doesn't make the grade for someone else—anyone else. Opinions will rain down on you like a hailstorm and much of it can be seriously hurtful.

I chose to write this book to reveal the muck and mire. It's not only healing for me, but for you too, the person who picks up this book and gets something out of it. Maybe you're encouraged to find sobriety and support. Maybe you know someone else who is suffering, and you'll have a better understanding of what they're enduring in their struggle. Maybe you will find the strength to reach out for help and heal, or gather the courage to tell your own story. Imagine a world in which we find the courage and freedom to tell our stories and help others.

If one person finds freedom, this book will be worth the time, effort, and soul-searching it took to get it written and published.

Are you struggling with alcohol, food, drugs, gambling, or sex? There is a solution and there are programs close by to help you. A boatload of people care and love you as you are, flaws and all. You don't have to live in that mess and space alone any longer—reach out for help.

Reach out to a friend you trust or a twelve-step program near you. Find peace for yourself and loosen the reins on the pressure you place on yourself about being perfect.

You don't have to know everything. I didn't. No one does.

A Story about Wrigley

Wrigley was a dog I adopted in the final months of my drinking. He is a powerful part of my journey and I want to tell his story as an illustration about how we can rise above and make the best of our choices, even when we aren't operating at optimum levels.

Most of what is below I posted on Facebook when I celebrated thirteen years of sobriety. Here's the story of my beloved dog, Wrigley, adapted from my post.

Thirteen years today of no drinking or drugging (January 13, 2022)! And today I want to share a part of my story in hopes it inspires one of you. In 2008 I moved to Jacksonville for my "dream" job of working with animals, but my life was anything but a dream. I was deep in the muck of drinking every single day and self-medicating so I would not have to face myself or life. I called in sick a lot during my probationary period of that job, and my performance on the job was less than adequate.

My job was doing field calls to help animals in need, and Wrigley was one of my last work rescue calls. He was an HBC—hit by car. When I arrived on the scene to pick him up, he was curled up under a bush, covered in a bloody road rash. But he was still wagging his tail, and he let me scoop him up and rush him to the shelter's vet. I knew there was something special about him.

Because he was a stray, he got put on hold to await his owner reclaiming him. In the meantime, I got "fired" for the pitiful display of what I thought was a stellar work performance. I

was furious—how dare they—and I did what any rational drunken, delirious person would do: I went and adopted that little oatmeal boy who had captured my heart.

So in October of 2008 I sat jobless, hopeless, and with my newly adopted dog. I proceeded to drink my life away, collecting unemployment. Drinking around the clock to numb myself wasn't cutting it, and I was spiraling out of control mentally and physically. By the end of December, family and friends were beginning to get concerned, and I knew deep within that something had to change.

By the grace of God, I was able to get into a detox center and with the support of a few trusted friends and family, I miraculously took my last drink and drug on 1/13/2009. Back then I never would have dreamed my life today would be running a farm sanctuary, rescuing animals, fundraising, marketing, and be so full of love and laughter with more friends and family than ever before.

Wrigley is super special on many levels, and he is one of the few things who is still a part of me and my past. He will always be part of my sober story. He helped me recover in those early days. I would never recommend adopting a dog when one's life is such a circus, but I did, and it proves that circumstances don't dictate the love and dedication that lies within. Together, over the past thirteen years, he and I have navigated life through homes, jobs, friends, cars, and the emotional ups and downs of living and getting sober. He is a forever friend, and I cannot imagine having had to walk that journey without him. Cheers to us both continuing to live healthy and happy lives together, one day at a time!

When Wrigley passed away, he ended an era of my sobriety. He was the last thing which had a direct connection to my days of drinking. He was a part of me before I got sober and stayed with me as a constant thread during my getting sober and learning a new way of life. His crossover from earth to spirit was a transition I never wanted to happen.

But the ebb and flow of life brings times of transition. Here is what I shared on social media with so many who grew to love him:

WRIGLEY, a teacher and friend to many, a magical gift to me.

October 2007–August 11, 2022

WRIGLEY will forever remain in our hearts!

His life was one to celebrate, and celebrating we did. After some Reiki, he enjoyed a fresh baked cake, had scrambled eggs for breakfast, and he got oodles of his favorite barn treat after doing the morning farm feedings with me.

He transitioned from the earth to spirit peacefully, with the help of a trusted veterinary friend and surrounded by those he loved.

I will cherish memories of him forever.

I miss his presence deeply, but I know that as time passes, that will lessen because I will rediscover his presence around me and stop looking for him where he once was.

He may no longer physically run to the barn every morning and night, but his energetic spirit lives on in the gardens and fields that surround us. May we all be blessed to know love as fiercely as Wrigley knew it and shared it with others.

If you have ever had any kind of pet, you will understand the love, bond, and commitment we pour into these creatures. For me, animals have always been a huge part of my life despite any addictions or life dilemmas. I knew from an early age I would not have children; I made this conscious choice because I had a deep-rooted drive to work with and help animals in need. And even within the chaos of my addiction I still stayed true to my inner calling, rescuing an animal, and I kept my commitment to Wrigley for his lifetime. It is a true testament that we have within us everything we need to overcome any challenges we face at any time.

Kody and the Pouch

How I Came to Stop Bingeing and Purging

I found myself standing in the bathroom, forty-two years young, staring at the toilet and ready to shove two fingers down my throat to purge the food I had binged on—another emotional bender of self-indulging comfort foods.

Three months earlier we'd moved to the farmhouse, and I'd sworn once we moved to my dream life, I would never engage in such self-destructive behavior again.

It was supposed to be a new beginning. Bulimia had been running my life for twenty-six years. Stopping completely was one of the biggest hurdles I had ever faced.

The all-too-familiar porcelain throne stared back at me. I was having a moment of clarity as I stood there reflecting on what I was doing, and my mind slowly catalogued the incident—the trigger—which had happened a few days prior.

We'd moved to the farmhouse to pursue my dream of rescuing horses and other farm animals. I was walking in the pasture with the newly arrived rescue horses. One of them bit me. Before that incident, I had respect for—but no fear of—horses. Our fostered horse changed things.

The trigger was *where* he bit me. He bit me right in my stomach area, the part of the belly where I had a thick layer of "fat" which I have never been able to get rid of. The pouch was the reason for

35

my many years of bingeing and purging. Trying to control and rid myself of that flab was my obsession.

Kody's bite caught me off guard and shook my confidence to the core. And yes, it hurt like crazy. Horses can nibble for attention or bite to get our attention. He was clearly making his position known and it was a bite.

Why is this pouch area so significant? It's the part of my stomach I have an intimate relationship with, one of love and hatred. I punched, poked, and stared in the mirror, making all kinds of weird contortions of that flab. It's a part of the belly I have battled—at peace with it one moment and royally hating it in the next.

Over time I've learned to love my pouch, but at that time of my life I despised it beyond words.

I've bought many workout tapes, watched, read, and listened to so many fitness trainers—who have seemingly flatter-than-flat stomachs—talk about how to get those flat, firm abs, but to no avail. Nope, it never happened for me.

The battle was daily, weekly, monthly, and yearly.

The battle of the bulging belly pouch went on for over twenty years, but one day, from an incident with a rescued horse named Kody, I gained a new perspective.

At the time, Kody was a foster horse. He and I were beginning to get acquainted. I was still green in living the farm life and taking care of horses. Little did he or I realize our relationship had taken on a new identity which would help not only me, but, eventually, others too.

During my decades of despising the pouch area, I would silently tell myself, as I completed yet another set of 100 abdominal crunches, maybe there was a reason I was unable to get rid of the pouch. Maybe said pouch was supposed to be there. Maybe it had a purpose. But I did not honor that area of my body other than having a random positive thought about it. I spent countless amounts of energy, money, and time hating it and trying desperately to get rid of it.

I resisted it endlessly.

So while my ego was bruised by the biting horse, those lingering effects of the bite surfaced in the bathroom that day.

As I stood ready to upchuck the food I had eaten, I thought, *Am I going to continue spending my time bingeing and purging after I've bought and created this farm to save, rescue, work with, and help animals in need? That's my true purpose and it's why I'm here—not to sit in a bathroom wasting time and energy abusing my body and soul.*

I had clarity so palpable I stood there in awe—a true aha moment. I don't have a journal entry recording the exact date I last binged and purged, but it was around March 2019, soon after the horses arrived, when Kody and I had that unforgettable encounter.

I remember the context of the day vividly. Kody was walking down the path, under the shade tree. We were having a bonding moment when, out of nowhere, he snapped his head around, bit me in the stomach, and ran off. He'd been at the farm for a couple of weeks, and we were still developing our relationship, learning how to respect one another and ultimately trust each other's presence.

As scary as the incident was, the bite didn't leave a mark on my belly. There was no bruising. There was no injury—other than to my ego and my self-confidence. The extra padding finally found its purpose.

The incident truly was a turning point in my self-image. It happened on the farm, at a time when I was following my desire to be with horses. It happened when I was slowly beginning to loosen the reins on the longtime pressure I'd put on myself and my life, and on the perceived high expectations from others.

I had finally let things go and followed my own path.

Twenty-six years of striving for perfection ... and I was finally able to see a purpose for the pouch which I felt had no business being part of me. The pouch was the cause of the delusional awareness I had about my image and outer appearance. It was the reason I binged and purged daily, sometimes multiple times a day. I sought refuge and solace in food and alcohol; overindulgence of a consumable "drug" made me instantly forget whatever I was facing.

Bingeing and purging allowed me to avoid my emotions.

I didn't know I was running from emotional pain. I thought it was the dang pouch and my need to please the world with a perfect body. I did of course get more attention from the boys and was liked by the cooler kids when I was thinner—at least it seemed that way.

Still, I was running from something emotionally. I was so fragile back in my teens and early twenties. Today I look back at that little girl and want to hug her and tell her how much she was loved and cared about by so many. It didn't matter what she looked like or how big or small her waistline was.

Can you relate? Do you know someone who is struggling like I did? Our paths might not be identical, but does the story sound familiar? Is food your best friend at times? Does indulging in sugary foods sound like a good idea, standing at the counter in the kitchen, in isolation? (Unless you have dogs, like I always did. Then you have eyes watching to see a crumb drop, which often happened.)

You're not alone, my friend. You are not alone. I understand the pain, and there is a way out.

The pouch still exists today. The difference is I have accepted it. And when I say accepted, I don't mean I am 100 percent okay with it. I accept it and don't fight it. I am more okay today with accepting my body as the body I was given, and I am okay with whatever shape and size my body chooses to be.

I love myself, my body included. I try to take good care of myself. You, too, can do that. I'm active, I eat healthily, I'm not sitting around eating bonbons and sucking down fatty fried foods anymore. I eat to fuel my body, and my body and soul are clean and in shape.

I'm thankful for strength today. Some days, acceptance is easier than others. Other times, it's barely enough to get through the day without being completely judgmental of myself. On those days I give myself grace and start anew the next day.

Esther Hicks, a spiritual teacher, medium, and guide, teaches when we stop resisting and pushing against that which isn't working for us, we'll see something wonderful happen. I look at the pouch as a part of me; it is my loving, unique shape and I have nothing to be ashamed of. If I look like everyone else, how am I unique? I want to be me and me only. I don't want to be you and have your body and your look. Your look is you, not me. There's a lot of peace and power with getting in touch with our own "perfection."

I've spent a great deal of time comparing myself to many other women and images that aren't even real. And honestly, who cares? I have no idea how someone gets to be the shape they are. For all I know, the person with the body I perceive as desirable is suffering behind closed doors with a raging eating disorder, and I most certainly don't want "that" body, if that's the cost! Or they might be unwell in any number of other ways.

Life is an adventure for each of us. It has taken me a long time to get to where I am: comfortable eating anything and everything, except my trigger foods, of course, and not thinking of purging.

I don't want to go back to feeling like I did when controlled by the bingeing and purging. I wasted countless hours and energy on planning the foods I would eat, how much, and when and where I could safely purge, every single time I ate. Numerous times, I started arguments because I couldn't get to a place to purge, or had to leave a party with friends and family early, only to find a place to go purge. It was pathetic.

But I won't beat myself up over it, and neither should you. It doesn't matter where you are on your journey. The experiences it takes to get where we are—where you are—are part of the process.

We can't get to where we want to be without going through where we have come. It took me time, patience with myself, learning from others, and listening to my inner spirit guide to shake free of the resistance.

Today I choose alignment with my wholeness and the love energy of who I am as an infinite being on this earth, with far more to express than what I look like. For me, getting in touch with being a beloved child of God is often a source of peace and strength beyond measure.

I have ended the resistance.

The Man in the Arena

I hope the stories and background I have already shared give you an idea of my history: when things started and how they have evolved.

Looking at our past and recognizing where we have come from is part of the process to recover, heal, and move forward. You certainly don't have to write about your life in a book, but finding someone to talk with about your past helps to get stuff out of your personal closet and clear the path for a brighter future. Think of it maybe as a good spiritual housecleaning.

Recovery is a pilgrimage. You will change, life will change around you, and the people in your life will change. It may not be easy and it may not feel like fun, but if you want a freer, more peaceful way of life, it will be worth going—and growing—through the changes and challenges.

I want to encourage and inspire you, yet please remember we each have our own path and no person's path is the same as another's.

The only way I've been able to choose abstinence of the eating disorder is that I was desperate to rise above the negative energy and to live a loving life. I had to choose a different response in my relationship with food, alcohol, and my body.

Despite sometimes feeling like a fraud—especially if I'm tired or hungry—and still battling with the thoughts in my scrambled mind, I've made peace with my body, no matter what size or shape it is at the moment. That doesn't mean those thoughts are gone forever and I've achieved this platform of healing, and I am better than anyone else. Goodness, no!

Heck, I've admitted I felt like a fraud writing this book, even as I poked my belly. But while I may still recognize that pouch, I choose to see it differently today.

This book serves as my platform for sharing the darkness with the light, the ugliness with the joy, so I can be completely transparent with you. That's where the magic happens. When we can relate to each other because we're not perfect, we find freedom. We give each other permission to not be perfect and to *be*—to be in self-awareness of what we are feeling and doing in the present.

None of it is good or bad or indifferent, it just *is*. We can acknowledge the thoughts and still choose to live with love and kindness—which starts with ourselves. Often this is referred to as choosing to live in the higher vibration of life and consciousness.

It's like making a conscious choice to choose the high road in life versus letting ego get in the way. We don't have to prove a point right or wrong in every situation.

Choosing the high road is kindness, and it emanates in everything from my relationship with my husband, job, pets, friends, family, food, and myself, and my body in particular. It takes practice to choose the right things in the various areas of our life. Sometimes it means simply stepping back and taking a break.

For instance, it's the moment when someone stole your parking spot in a full parking lot, you had to park far away, and you refrained from saying or doing something foolish due to the fact that you knew "it was your spot."

That's ego poking us, and we can take a deep breath, put on a smile, and let ego go on by. We can choose, moment by moment, to take the high road. Like I said earlier, it does take practice, but I've found by keeping at it, it becomes automatic.

I want you to understand we're all human. Some days it'll seem easier to find peace and be kind than on other days. We get stronger by being tested. We have strengths and flaws, easier days and harder ones. But if I can do this, I want you to know that if you want to, you can, too.

There's no right or wrong here, only what works best for each of us. Each reader is going to take something different from this book, and I encourage you to allow yourself permission to take what resonates with you and leave the rest.

I've already achieved one goal. Writing this book has helped me. I can hope it helps you too—even if only to offer you a little hope. I may not do things precisely the way someone else deems they should have been done, but I get up and participate in life—it's the only way!

There is a famous quote by Theodore Roosevelt that I reference often. Have you ever heard of "The Man in the Arena"? An excerpt follows:

> It is not the critic who counts; not the man who points out how the strong man stumbles, or where the doer of deeds could have done them better. The credit belongs to the man who is actually in the arena, whose face is marred by dust and sweat and blood; who strives valiantly; who errs, who comes short again and again, because there is no effort without error and shortcoming; but who does actually strive to do the deeds; who knows great enthusiasms, the great devotions; who spends himself in a worthy cause; who at the best knows in the end the triumph of high achievement, and who at the worst, if he fails, at least fails while daring greatly, so that his place shall never be with those cold and timid souls who neither know victory nor defeat.

Our humaneness will always be challenged by ego, but I am learning I don't have to serve my ego. I can let my ego propel me forward and use it to do good. It can serve me.

Think about having your fist wrapped around something so tight you can't let it go. We hold ourselves hostage when we're in the scarcity mentality. Dr. Wayne W. Dyer says, in many of his recordings, "You can either be a host to God or a hostage to your ego."

I am perfect the way I am. And I love my perfect imperfection.

And I hope you will love yours, too!

Freedom and peace mean I'm not bound to conform to what society deems perfect. And one way I have finally decided to no longer conform is to step out and follow my true heart's passion.

I stepped into the arena of my own life when I followed a calling I always had on my heart and soul.

Listening to the Call

Have you always known there's something deeper, something more meaningful you're supposed to be doing? Like a calling on your soul you can feel and hear. Over time the calling gets louder as you navigate through life. But that noise within is something we ignore because society and others tell us it isn't real—or isn't important.

I've always known I have a gift for animals. And the knowledge grew deeper as I grew older. It became more real and evident the more I gave it an opportunity to come alive by deciding to follow the call to work with animals.

Although I knew I had gifts and a calling, I never knew how my calling would play out in life.

> We all have gifts and talents. The magic is in discovering what those are for each of us.

For forty-four years I ignored the calling of my heart and soul, until I gathered the courage to finally listen and step off on my own. Sharing my story and how I came to step onto my own path is part of that calling. And the personal brand of #BeKind has been the greatest inspiration to my path.

Kody the horse taught me to be kind. And, in giving Kody up and giving up my insecurities and asking for the kind of training we both needed, I discovered kindness is part of acceptance, too. Be Kind to yourself, each other, and those around you—people, animals, and the planet.

For many of you, reading this book is the first time we're meeting. While I'm the author, I'm also the founder of an education farm sanctuary and organization whose mission is to inspire compassion, as mentioned earlier.

While abstinence from an eating disorder fueled me to write this book, the rescued animals are the foundation *for* the book. They have already inspired me to write and illustrate several children's books. This memoir is my first adult book and hopefully the beginning of more to come.

My dream has always been to have a cow or a horse of my own, but I was always so consumed by my own pity party, I never focused long enough to even consider the dream might be possible.

When I was addicted to drinking and bingeing and purging, I would sit on bar stools solving world problems and contemplating how I would save the world and all the animals, but I could never stay sober long enough to make anything become a reality.

When I finally got sober, the dream I had buried deep within slowly began to surface. Living with clarity of mind made me realize it wasn't a dream, but a calling. I couldn't avoid the call, no matter how hard I tried.

And trust me, I tried. Like the story of Jonah who said no to God's calling and ended up in the belly of the whale, I said "no" through my lifestyle of addictions.

Over time, in my walk of getting sober I took steps toward making the dream—the calling—become a reality.

In 2015 I started EPIC Outreach, a nonprofit 501(c)(3) organization, with a goal to create an education farm sanctuary where rescued animals could share their stories, which inspire kindness and compassion.

I had never owned a horse, I had never taken riding lessons, I didn't grow up on a farm, I knew nothing about what it meant to care for a horse or run a farm. I started researching, and learned as much as I could on my own. Over time and through lots of hours volunteering and asking so many questions of others who were more experienced than I was, I learned a lot.

In 2019 my husband, Jack, and I bought a seven-acre farm, and the sanctuary came to life.

The whole odyssey to creating one of the most magical places on the planet has taught me much about myself. It's still teaching me things about slowing down, dropping perfection, and centering myself so I can listen to the energies of life and flow rather than force things into submission. I feel like I'm reborn and living a life beyond my wildest dreams.

Today, at the time of the publication of this book, I'm in my mid-forties, running a rescue with fifty plus rescued animals who call the sanctuary home. I'm fortunate to engage with kids and adults, and to teach kindness and inspire compassion weekly, monthly, and yearly.

It *is* magical.

Along with creating the sanctuary, revealing my story through this book has been part of that calling.

It began with the encounter with Kody. I not only realized I needed to work with that horse on the ground to gain his respect, but the turning point was when I found myself in my routine of being alone in the house and still resorting to bingeing and purging.

Kody gave me a wake-up call. I love food and I love to eat, but I would overindulge, especially when I didn't know how to control the things happening around me.

Isn't that what humans often do?

We avoid the things which cause us pain or discomfort by replacing them with other things, which are usually self-destructive behaviors like drinking, drugs, gambling, sex, or bingeing and purging.

In the pink bathroom of the farmhouse one day, I stood there over the toilet, staring into the mirror and realizing I could be spending my time in the pasture with the animals, building a relationship with the horses I so desperately craved.

And it was not that I *could* be—I *wanted* to be there.

I'd created the farm sanctuary so I had the space and time to do good, and here I was wasting time in a cycle I'd been living for twenty-seven years of my life.

I've learned that human beings hold on to the things we know, which keeps us stuck in the places we no longer want to be.

So, at one pivotal moment in the bathroom, I made a choice. I took a stand. "No more." Three months into living at the farmhouse, I drew a line in the sand.

That day in the bathroom was the first day of my abstinence.

Compare and Contrast

My entire quality of life shifted when I began to be kind to myself. I've always been one to seek a better way of living, thinking, and doing things. I want to learn how to be a better steward of the planet, a better steward of my body, of my mind, of the relationships in my life, of my money, and of the things that surround me.

Yes, a big shift began when I got sober, but a truly authentic shift began when I started listening to the voice within and followed the voice—my inner calling.

We all have an inner voice, a spiritual guidance which directs us through feelings, ideas, and impulses. It takes time to learn what the dialogue sounds like and align with that inner voice. Sometimes the external noises are way louder, and it can be challenging to navigate through the noise. The voices on the outside are influenced by the external world and can be deafening.

I found a place of acceptance and learned to stop listening to the external noises.

The learning took time and practice. I can easily get caught up in the external voice when I compare myself to others. I've been notorious for fixating on what *others* look like. I'd ask them how they stayed so thin—and when I say fixate, I mean fixate.

I'd obsess over how someone dressed, comparing how a piece of clothing looked on one person versus how it would or did look on me. I'd watch what people ate or drank and took inventory on how much they consumed, romanticizing I might be able to eat what they ate without any repercussions.

I'd compare my legs, abs, butt, arms, chin, and neck to those of others.

It took a long time to unravel that comparison trait.

It took constant reminders from a mentor who called me out when I compared myself to others. In my work to accept and love my body image, I had to learn while I am *like* others, I'm *not* others. She always said, "You are not comparing apples to apples. Look at your path and look at the unknown path of the other person. You don't know their journey or struggles, or even what they struggle with today, right now as we speak, so you cannot do that comparison."

And she was right. I don't know if the person eating goes and purges or starves themselves for days to be able to eat like that. I don't know what size clothing they're wearing. It's about perception. If I perceive a person is wearing a size "small" doesn't mean it's a fact. They could be wearing a size "large" which looks like a size "small" to me. All this evaluation is an exhausting use of mental power.

While the message to not compare was drilled into my brain hundreds of times, the lack of confidence and low self-esteem I've always harbored led me to repeated comparisons. I didn't trust myself.

Striving for what society tells us is perfection comes at a huge price. For some people, it comes at the ultimate price. For me, the price of comparison was restriction, starvation, bingeing and purging, and self-hatred. When I compare myself to you and others around me, I'm not *only* judging you, but I'm judging you—and me—unfairly. Comparing apples to oranges isn't a comparison and is most likely what I was doing. The truth is, I have no idea what anyone else is dealing with. But to some extent, many of us do this throughout our lifetime. We judge one another about all sorts of things.

Do we actually have any idea what internal and external battles a stranger is facing? Do we even know their age, background, or what they've done to get where they are today? Quite frankly, it's none of our business.

It took the repetition of reprogramming myself to get past the self-ridicule. I had to experience awakenings which allowed me to recognize when my internal voice was making comparisons. I could then make a conscious choice to dismiss the judgments and free myself of the cycle of self-condemnation.

Did this happen overnight? No way. It takes time and consistency to change a pattern of doing, thinking, and believing things that don't empower us.

I began to practice shifting my thoughts as I became aware of those harmful thoughts in different scenarios.

I'm going to share a few of those with you.

Voices in My Head

Comparing myself to others was a fixation and so were the voices in my head.

My mind has conversations with itself, and I must be vigilant to stop and remind myself not to fixate on things the voices in my head are saying; often those are lies. Our minds can help or hurt us!

If you have a brain like mine that never stops, it can make for a long life of misery. But when we recognize our brain will always think and always conjure things up, we can train ourselves to think differently in order to act and react differently.

January 28, 2019, was a sad day. And it provided an aha moment regarding the lies my brain could tell.

I woke up to find little Pumpkin had passed away overnight.

Pumpkin was a guinea pig EPIC Outreach had rescued and saved from the brink of death in 2016. She was the cutest little thing, with swirls of long orange, white, and brown hair. She squeaked loudly when it was feeding time, eager to sink her teeth into a carrot or leafy green veggie. As an education ambassador, for several years she visited classrooms in many schools, after-school programs, and summer camps. She truly was an integral part of fulfilling the mission of EPIC Outreach. She was popular with many kids and adults.

Pumpkin wasn't feeling well the day before I found her lifeless body. I'd planned to take her to the vet that morning, but it was too late. I'll be honest: at first it didn't register. I had to go look at her lifeless body in her cage several times. I picked her up and held her close.

It was sad. It was scary.

After I let it sink in, I fell apart. I crawled onto my bed and gazed out the window overlooking the backyard, as I often did to pray. I stared out into the sky through the tree branches, and a voice—the bloody judgmental inner voice spoke up—the one in my head which screams the loudest at my weakest moments.

And I was in the middle of one of those weak moments.

I heard it yelling, *"You are terrible. You should have taken her to the vet yesterday. You call yourself a rescuer? Look at this—you can't even save your guinea pig. Guinea pigs can live to be eight years of age and she barely made it four years."*

The energy work I'd been doing made me sure enough of myself to tell the voice to shut the bleep up! I reaffirmed to myself the voice might be there, but I didn't have to listen to it. That voice was not truth. It was after me in this time of need and sorrow, in my vulnerability. I had to dig deep to remind myself, *I'm a good pet parent. I do good for all things.*

Having power over those negative voices in our minds is about reprogramming our mental responses. I amazed myself that morning. Ordinarily, I'd have let the voice take me out of the game and send me into a spiraling internal self-attack.

At that moment I knew I had a choice to disrupt those voices in my head. Was their message one of loving myself? It was not, and that's our first clue. Those negative messages are always there and they're always out to get us. It's up to us to either cater to them, or discount them and move on. It's taken me a lot of practice to learn that skill. Believe me, sometimes those voices are louder than I prefer.

I've often wondered if it would be nice to have a volume regulator to turn down those voices when they get out of control. Or maybe install an internal mute button.

By way of these kinds of life situations, we get to practice self-control and self-love. Through using the reprogramming and rewiring I've learned about being worthy of love and kindness, how I respond to life and its events is up to me. I'm free to live my most desired life as my most authentic self.

Who Let the Dogs Out?

Another example of the voices happened one Friday night. It was 5:30 p.m. and I'd come in from saying hello to the farm animals. My husband had gone off to a concert, which left me to care for the dogs inside the house. They required feeding and letting them out to go potty. At the time, we had five inside dogs.

The day had been stormy, with lots of rain.

When I got inside, there was a lull in the rain. I was in my office cleaning things up before I began the ritual of feeding the hungry hounds. As I finished what I was doing, a torrential downpour let loose.

Immediately, the voice in my head got on me. *You should have let the dogs out first. Now they won't go out.* Of course, this made sense. I don't know about you, but if you have dogs like mine, they each turn into a poodle the moment it begins to get wet outside and they don't want to get their dainty Rottweiler and pit bull paws wet.

I was hard on myself instantly, as if I was supposed to be perfect at everything. The banter in my head continued. *You should have taken them out first.*

You dummy, now you have to wait to let them out, which means you have to wait to feed them. You can't feed them and not let them out.

On and on went the ridiculing thoughts. But right after they started running through my head, I remembered growing up being ridiculed for not doing "something right." I could almost *feel* my childhood struggle to be perfect.

In the dog scenario, I chose to clean my office, it happened to rain, and I had to wait to feed the dogs before letting them out.

I've been mentored to look at the facts and the "what is" of the moment. No "shoulds" allowed. Stick to the facts: I was cleaning my room and it rained. Simple. I didn't need to ridicule myself for something like rain. Rain was out of my control. I didn't know torrential rain would resume before I'd gotten the dogs fed.

My mentor says, "Give it back." Those negative thoughts are not kind or loving. I'm not allowed to own ridicule of myself. I must give it back to my childhood and choose to be kind to myself.

The internal self-talk and ridicule, time after time, will start to sink in and we end up with tons of negative self-talk that we start to believe. It doesn't have to be ridiculing our character, though. Maybe the voice wants to convince us we don't have enough of something and, because we have a false belief of lack, we want to hang on to things we don't need.

That was me when we moved to the farmhouse. I had stuff everywhere. I got comfortable in my life and many things piled up, finding their way into corners and crevices of the house. Things were tucked wherever I could find a place to put them. I became aware I was holding on to belongings, not willing to let anything go.

I think it was based in a fear of missing out or not having enough.

When I mustered up the courage to finally drop stuff off at the thrift store—after painfully coming to terms with letting it go—I drove around with it in my car for days, or weeks, with the intention of dropping it off. But I still felt the need to "hold on," doubtful that I was finally willing to let it go.

Even after I'd made the concrete decision to pull into the parking lot of the store to unload, I double-checked the box to make sure everything in there was what I wanted to donate. Is this worth money? Am I letting go of something that someone else is going to make a million dollars on? Talk about a headache!

A few days ago, I found the same belongings tucked away in a closet and I didn't even know it was there until I started to clean that closet. And most of the stuff was previously someone else's to begin with. I'm a thrift store shopper. Jeesh, another exhausting cycle.

But my mentors taught me well. What is the truth of the situation? I realized I needed to Let. It. Go! And I needed to tell the voices to be quiet.

The situation itself doesn't matter; those voices are always there, ready to rear their ugliness and rob us of our power and joy. We need to stay vigilant to keep the voices in their place.

Those Voices and Writing

I've always loved to write, and the ideas and creativity that flow in and through my mind and soul are incredible. Constant, really. But the smallest things can challenge my self-confidence and take me out of the game I know I'm here to play.

Writing, the thing I love, can be a trigger that challenges my self-worth when I compare myself to others.

I could easily go into a mental orbit when I saw one friend comment on another friend's social media post. They'd asked that friend, "When are you going to write a book?"

Where did *my* brain go?

Hmmm, no one has said that to me. Why hasn't anyone asked me that question? I love to write, and I like to think my writing is engaging and fun and tells a good story.

I looked for a way to soothe my emotions and turned to food. I'd go get a bag of my favorite snack chips and eat my feelings away. That *one* comment on that *one* post on that *one* friend's timeline on social media could distract me from my fullest potential.

What. The. Heck!

I'm not kidding about this. Our minds are the craziest things. They can take us out of the game of life or keep us in it. It's up to us to choose what thoughts we'll think and how we'll allow them to direct our lives.

With the writing, I worked diligently to stop comparing myself to others and I got quiet. I went within and prayed to the universe for a new thought. My inner guide told me, *Those who succeed in what they are passionate about don't wait for the sales or the wins to come to them, they go after it.*

I knew if I was committed to accomplishing the things I know are my path, like writing and the mission of EPIC Outreach, then I would have to stop listening to the negative voices. I had to follow the positive energy and watch what happened.

That might sound foo-foo and airy-fairy to some, but it made sense. I've experienced this truth.

I follow the guidance within. I listen to the internal voice which is loving and encouraging. I trust all things are working out when I stay true to that path.

I know I'm here to be a light and sharer of love for the planet. When I can quiet my mind and stop the negative voices, I'm able to let the inner tempo guide me. The negative voices in my head get quieter the longer and the more I practice not listening to them, and instead choose the more positive voice, thoughts, and feelings to align with.

I'm strong, smart, and capable. I'm a person who can choose the thoughts I think and the feelings I feel. You also have this ability. Our Creator has given us gifts, and missions, and provides the loving guidance to make us successful with them.

When you want something bad enough, you'll go to any lengths to get it.

It's possible to shift from negative to positive. Get a mentor who is positive and knowledgeable and loving. Surround yourself with positive people.

With the support of good people who taught me good things, I began to choose positive thoughts and I could stop fixating on other people.

A Spiritual Path: Alcoholics Anonymous

Connecting to our innermost selves is a spiritual activity. I've learned to recognize those voices in my head and seek counsel from the spirit which guides and directs me from within. Some might call that spirit guide the Holy Spirit, or God, or their higher power. We have that connection built in, but we only have access to it—can only hear it—when we are humble enough to ask for it.

I got disconnected from my internal guidance system when I was drinking, and bingeing and purging. I reconnected to my spiritual self after getting sober.

There's a saying that we are spiritual beings having a human experience, and I believe to my deepest core that saying is true.

Alcoholics Anonymous (AA) is a program of recovery which has been a huge cornerstone in my personal recovery and the shaping of my spiritual journey. AA has a 12-step program, and the 11th step is one of my favorites.

What is Step 11 of AA? "Sought through prayer and meditation to improve our conscious contact with God as we understood God, praying only for knowledge of God's will for us and the power to carry that out."

The 11th step embodies our conscious contact with a power greater than us. I love that so much. Out of this exercise, I started EPIC Outreach, the nonprofit with a focus on raising people's consciousness to make more compassionate choices in life for people, animals, and the planet.

Raising my own consciousness was part of my solution to getting sober and staying abstinent. And it's in direct alignment with what I'm doing in the world through and with EPIC Outreach.

When I was growing up in New Jersey, we went to church every Sunday. My dad never went, but my mom was involved as a deacon at the Presbyterian church. My mom was part of the fellowship of that church, doing a lot with members of the church, in it and outside of it.

While I attended Sunday school as a kid, I don't remember understanding who God was and what spirituality was. I enjoyed being in a classroom or sitting in the pews with my mom when we attended the adult services. I have fond memories learning about God, church life, and that Jesus loves me, but anything deeper is vague.

Moving around with my father's job from New Jersey to Texas to Germany made attending church inconvenient. During those moves we stopped going to church. I had an understanding of who God was, I knew he existed, and I had my Bible, but I didn't know a thing about being *spiritual*.

During my high school years we didn't go to church, but I knew how to pray. I did the ol' foxhole prayers whenever I was in trouble or found myself drinking, drugging, and bingeing and purging.

God, I promise to do better if you help me.

God, if you help me get out of this I will start doing __ ....

God was like Santa Claus in the sky.

It wasn't until I got into a program of recovery that I learned more about God. When I came into the program of AA I was reintroduced to spirituality. At first, the mention of God in the meetings would make my skin crawl, so much that I wanted to get up and walk out. But a sponsor taught me to stay seated and grow where my feet were planted.

I went into the rooms of AA primarily due to my drinking, but also for my raging eating disorder. I've already said that eating disorders are something which few people talk about; the subject gets swept under the carpet. I've been getting more comfortable talking about it the longer I stay abstinent and the more grounded I am in my spiritual growth. The more comfortable I get with myself, the more I want to disclose the story of overcoming a battle so fierce, I once thought that battle and I were hopeless.

I came into a program of recovery because either my drinking or my bulimia had to stop first, and I chose to end the abuse of alcohol before I addressed the eating disorder. My addictions were out of control and had me on a path to death, jail, or an institution.

I needed a spiritual intervention.

What is spirituality, anyway? God, Jesus, the Holy Spirit, or all three? I never understood it fully. If you're like me and don't understand it, don't worry. All you need to do is believe in something bigger than you. Stop worrying about the political correctness of what *you* call it.

I may have offended a few of you. While that wasn't my intention, it's okay. We live in a nation in which we're free to believe anything we want. If what or who you believe in works for you and what I believe in works for me, and we are both living a life of conscious awareness, doesn't everyone win?

Don't let your concept of spirituality be the block to your healing. Don't let your ego use that as an excuse to keep you captive! You don't have to believe in God, but you will have to believe in something greater than you. I believe in God. For others it's the universe, and some believe it's the energy within the world such as a table, a doorknob, a pet cat, or the flowers and trees.

Everything is energy: the table, the book you're holding, the digital device you're reading or listening on, the pen I wrote this book with. It's all energy vibrating in harmony with you and everything around you.

There's an energy within this world that's always guiding and directing us.

I needed to tap into that spiritual energy to launch my healing.

I've mentioned God a few times and I've mentioned the universe a few times. I believe there's energy within the universe, vibrating in everything. Universal energy guides me, through my inner being. I've learned to hear it and understand. That universal energy guides me through the things God has placed in my heart—those things I desire and dream of. I get creatively inspired. A collective of intentions and energy guides me.

Just as I've applied a spiritual program to getting sober, I have dug even deeper to find spiritual alignment within my body. Working with the energies for my body has provided me with many discoveries. To uncover those misalignments has meant making peace with my body, making peace with my soul, and seeing spirit and my body as friends.

Connecting with my body and talking to it builds on that connection. I've learned to ask my body, "What do you want?"

"What do you need?"

Nine times out of ten, it says *"An apple"* when my brain tells me I want pretzels. I know if I follow the guide, I am good; but if I follow my fleshly ways and eat the pretzels, I'm doomed.

Will it kill me? No, but I self-sabotage and resent myself because I didn't listen to the spirit within which will *always* guide me to the highest and best action. It took me a long time to understand that and trust it. I often want to question what my internal guides are saying.

We can easily make stuff up to change the messages, especially if it results in getting what our negative self wants. I had to get to a place where I accepted that fact and decided to stand firm in the belief. We're either going to trust this guidance or we aren't.

Learning to listen to the internal guidance has been a process that has affected the choices I make: from which foods to eat, starting a rescue education farm sanctuary, to trusting the message urging me to write my book.

At one point, one of the messages I heard was: *If you don't write the book, I will ask someone else with a similar experience. So take the time to share your story. It needs to be heard.*

There is a story about a football player who was given a multimillion-dollar contract to play a sport. He was spiritually connected and received a message to go be a farmer.

What?

Stop playing football, give up the money, fame, and security to be a farmer?

He had no idea how to farm. He had to teach himself, using YouTube videos, about everything from running a tractor to planting seeds. His mission for the farm was to provide produce to help people less fortunate in the community. He was successful and still is today. In interviews, he says his life is more fulfilling than it would have been if he'd stayed on the path of money and fame as a pro football player.

His name is Jason Brown, of First Fruits Farm. I invite you to look up his inspiring story.

Our job is not to figure out the how or the why. Our job is to listen, trust, and follow the guidance we're given.

The Pandemic – COVID-19

For twenty-seven years I used food to fuel my actions and control my emotional reactions, by regulating how much I ate and how much of that I allowed my body to keep. That self-hating lifestyle finally came to a halt when I bought our seven-acre farm and began to work with horses and other rescued farm animals.

As I said earlier, I've started and stopped this memoir for years. I started writing initially in 2019, when I began to write my thoughts on paper. I jotted things down or stored them in my mind—letting them collect dust on shelves in my office and in my brain. That procrastination went on for a year, and in 2020 the COVID-19 pandemic happened.

That incident flipped the world upside down and gave the *Loosen the Reins* manuscript a whole new perspective.

The following words are from what I journaled during the pandemic. I am sure you will find many similarities to what you experienced and witnessed during that period.

The coronavirus, or COVID-19 (how it will be referred to), was a rapidly spreading virus with no cure at the time of this writing, and it started in one country, spreading like wildfire through humans. It was passed on in a similar way as the flu, with lots of sneezing, coughing, unwashed hands, infected doorknobs, and transference of the virus to the face.

The virus came to the public's awareness after it surfaced in China, after the New Year of 2020. It quickly increased its reach through people traveling abroad. While China was the first to report massive endemic infections and deaths, Italy quickly followed, reporting a complete lockdown of its citizens. A lockdown meant everyone had to stay at home to prevent the health systems from being overloaded since they were already compromised by everyday illnesses and other medical needs. The World Health Organization (WHO) got involved to help the world manage health information, medical and research breakthroughs, and global statistics.

The United States government began sharing information and heavily emphasized the importance of washing our hands. In March the US realized that beating this horribly deadly virus would take more than guiding people to wash their hands. The World Health Organization announced that the world was indeed in the clutches of a pandemic, and US news broadcasts began talking of ways to "flatten the curve," which was a term used to refer to preventing something from growing or increasing in a small amount of time.

One way to do that was to begin social distancing and that quickly became the number one weapon against the spread. Strong measures were advised by government officials, the WHO, and a variety of medical experts desperate to stop the spread and deaths. It quickly became the thing spoken about around the clock on every news station, all over social media, and in print. Social distancing meant to keep six feet between one another. That included keeping our distance from family, friends, colleagues, and others we might encounter while out in the community—when we were allowed to be outside our homes.

In two months, social distancing became the norm.

It was advised to stay at home unless necessary, like going to a doctor's visit, picking up groceries or medications, taking your pet to the vet, and so on. It felt like overnight we went from a functioning society where just about anything was allowed, to a complete halt in almost every aspect of life.

Everyone was asked to wear a mask over their mouth and nose if they were outside their home, and personal protective equipment (PPE) became a new buzz word.

Life as we knew it drastically changed. Some of the things listed below became "normal" for many.

- Schools were ordered closed, many of which were already on spring break; they were not going to return until at least May, if at all, for the rest of the school year.

- Virtual learning was implemented in a matter of weeks.

- Businesses were asked to have employees work from home and only essential workers were to report to places of work.

- Tape was placed on the floors at grocery stores and other places people visited to help distance shoppers six feet from one another.

- Limits were placed on the number of people allowed inside stores, causing lineups outside store doors and in parking lots.

- Nonessential stores and businesses were mandated to close.

- Parks, beaches, and some public entities were closed until further notice.

- Large theme parks like Disneyland, SeaWorld, and Aquatica were closed.

- Entire sports seasons were canceled, to include the National Basketball Association playoffs, the Professional Golfers Association Tour, and Major League Baseball.

- Concerts, tours, festivals, and entertainment events were canceled.

- Weddings, family celebrations, holiday gatherings were canceled.

- Gatherings of more than fifty people were banned, and

that number was quickly reduced to no more than ten people.

- We realized a shortage of masks, gowns, and gloves for frontline and emergency workers.

- There was a shortage of ventilators for the critically ill.

- Panic buying set in, and we had no toilet paper, no disinfecting supplies, no paper towels, no laundry soap, and no hand sanitizer.

- Shelves were bare of certain items during times of hurricane preparedness.

- The government closed the border to all nonessential travel.

- Fines were established for breaking the rules, some tracking compliance via cell phone / tower information.

- Press conferences were issued daily from the president, which included updates on new cases, recoveries, and deaths.

- Formerly jammed roadways were nearly empty.

- People wore masks everywhere, some even wore gloves. In a wide variety, mask designs were made at home, in dress shops, or available online and in stores.

- Home delivery of groceries, other foods, and beverages became a new industry.

- Millions of people were laid off and/or lost their jobs. If we were lucky enough to remain employed, we were grateful.

- Restaurants were closed for indoor dining; eventually, take-out and delivery were available.

It was a scary time for many. Being required to shelter in place for an indefinite time frame had many people going a little stir-crazy. Politicians became unempathetic, crashing under pressure as they scrambled to heal the economy, increase lifesaving, and end the virus that was robbing the world of safety, security, health, and wealth.

I kept thinking that this might be the planet screaming for a reset. It was like the universe was asking for everyone to slow down, stop the crazy pace we all seemed to keep, and look at how things could be done differently. Could it be a time of healing for the people, the earth, and communities around the globe?

When things came to a screeching halt like they did, it made people across the world slow down and stop the hustle and bustle of life. There were images of the normally busy bumper-to-bumper eight-lane Los Angeles freeways empty of traffic. The streets of New York City were quiet, with not a soul in sight. Airlines accustomed to flying two million passengers to destinations everywhere were down to 100,000 passengers traveling for the entire year.

Those things were an indication that the world—humanity—probably needed an enormous healing.

I knew it applied to me.

As did so many others, I felt the nudge to slow down and reevaluate my life.

I had already started the process of healing within, but those times advanced my healing. Did you listen to the external messages at that time? Did you turn inward to look at where things might need to slow down for you?

COVID-19 altered so many lives, whether you knew someone directly affected with the virus or indirectly affected. People had a loved one suffer a stroke, and because of COVID-19 these folks couldn't go visit them in the hospital to support them.

Imagine this: We could only visit our husbands, dads, or children via virtual meeting calls while they lay in a hospital bed. Zoom became the go-to online platform for communicating with those we couldn't see in person in a hospital or at a jobsite.

That kind of disconnection affected our lives emotionally and psychologically, and probably will for generations to come.

Many people passed away from COVID-19, and families were not permitted to have a funeral to say their final goodbyes or get together to celebrate their loved one's life and legacy. The lack of normal closure has lasting effects on a griever's soul.

When we stop to listen to the messages from the universe, the world, the planet, we are guided. In those moments the real song and dance with life begins. Since my life was already on a path of awakening when COVID-19 occurred, the pandemic was the fuel my soul needed to get active pursuing that dream and the path placed in my heart many years earlier.

The intense emotions and weight of the pandemic lit the fire for me to assemble those many scraps of paper and ideas and write *Loosen the Reins*. I had chosen the title in 2019, after beginning the adventure of creating the education farm sanctuary. I had no idea of the significant effect the farm sanctuary would have on me and my eating disorder recovery. Over the course of a year, during 2019–2020, my spirit was molded and refined by the daily interaction of large spiritual animals.

I picked up the pace of completing the memoir in March 2020, amid COVID-19. That was also a time when I started learning and adopting the teachings of Esther Hicks. Abraham's teachings taught me a deeper understanding of higher-level energy work and how to focus my attention on being joyful rather than worrying about the things I didn't have or couldn't control.

The pandemic gave me the perfect opportunity to slow down and pivot in my life.

During the pandemic I took paid time off from work. While everyone was social distancing, I soaked up the outdoors with

Kody, Taz, Buck, Zimba, Zeke, Oliver, and Tator, the rescued farm animals. I fired up the pen and fingertips to get the writing done. I had about 13,200 words to begin, and after some research I realized I needed about 50,000 more for a decent memoir. So began the writing process, a labor of love.

Even with those best intentions, scheduled paid time off, and the required slowdown by a world pandemic, the same internal challenges I had faced years ago kept popping up. I will let any distraction be more important than writing, when the thing I have been praying for and asking to do with my life is to write.

But writing this memoir meant I had to get real and vulnerable when putting my thoughts to paper, and I avoided it at all costs. So while I say the book has been a real *joy* to write, it has caused me lots of anxiety too. I confess this to be fully transparent.

It is like this: I set a goal to take time off to get something done—writing—and somehow everything else comes up. The dog needs a bath and its nails trimmed, the barn needs to be organized, I must paint my nails, I need to plant a garden, the dust that has collected all year must be wiped away today, and the list goes on ad infinitum. Before I knew it, my time off was gone and I hadn't even started what I set out to accomplish.

I always put my best intentions forth, and yet I seem to find ways to sabotage them.

Every. Single. Time.

I asked myself, *Am I avoiding the task of writing or is it something more?*

After years of doing self-discovery work, I have learned to look inward on these things. Oftentimes I find it's not the task that I'm avoiding, but something deeper. The task is often about me *proving* myself and if I fail at that task, then I am a failure, right?

Many of us have a long-underlying root within us which says we have to prove we are worthy, that we are good enough. Perhaps it goes back to the people-pleasing thing: we always listened to what others had to say and didn't stand up for our beliefs.

The underlying root peaked for me during the writing of this book. Lots of self-doubt popped up. And self-doubt is the driving force behind trying to prove myself. My lack of confidence drove and can still drive me to push myself. The thoughts persisted: *Who would want to read this? You have nothing anyone else wants to hear or read. You aren't popular enough to write a book. No one will care what you have to say.* And on and on.

While our calling and God-driven direction might be to write a book, we'll often find other things to do instead.

Like let's check on social media. That's important! How many likes did we get on a post or how many followers do we now have on Instagram?

What animal can I rescue today?

Instead of writing the book, I wanted to focus on things like programs for the nonprofit. If I took time to stop and focus on writing, would I be missing out on capitalizing on the thing I wanted most—to prove I can be successful?

When social distancing started, social media revealed that everyone panicked about fundraising for nonprofits, small businesses closed, and people lost jobs. However, I wasn't in fear financially.

I was trying to figure out how I could get ahead and come up with some genius idea which would skyrocket my nonprofit and put it on the map. How could I leverage the downtime and changing priorities to help grow our nonprofit?

How was I going to become famous and get the pats on the back for my success and prove I knew what I was doing? Crazy, right?

People were dying and getting sick—a world pandemic—and I was trying to figure out how to be successful instead of slowing down and seeing how I could help someone else. My self-worth seemed to depend almost entirely on proving that I was credible.

And while emotional warfare waged in my mind and spirit, I knew enough at that stage of my journey to pray and quiet my mind in meditation.

I was listening, following, and implementing the teachings of Abraham, through Esther Hicks. Abraham is a collective consciousness which teaches the human realm through Esther Hicks. Those teachings resonate with me, and I've learned that when I get still and consult my inner self, the answer always comes to me. Then it's up to me to listen to the answer. And the answer was: *You are enough!*

I suspect the answer for many of us is that we are enough! And we are good enough: worthy of success, good health, good friends, and we have an admirable purpose. What we are doing is enough. Stop trying to do what others are doing, stop trying to compete, stop trying to prove ourselves.

If you want to do something that's in your heart, do it, but do it because you're inspired to do it, not because you want to prove something or be successful.

Since I started this project, I've learned from professional writers that putting our writing last on the to-do list is not uncommon. Some even joke about sometimes finding themselves cleaning toilets and scrubbing floors instead of writing.

A Drive for Perfection

During COVID-19, the groups I followed and learned from were posting great virtual ideas for engagement with followers and how to invite new followers and supporters. Online engagement became everything when virtual contact was all anyone had available.

I had ideas rolling around in my head too, but I didn't reveal them. Instead I posed a question on social media, asking people to respond with feedback. I was terrified to post my ideas. If they failed, I'd look like I didn't know what I was doing. In my mind, there wouldn't be anything worse.

The groups I perceived as successful had the commitment and confidence to post what they were committed to. They trusted that the audience and support would show up, and if it didn't, they would adjust. I was committed to my creation, but lacked confidence. However, I was learning there's no need to ask permission. Do it and trust that the right people—whether the number is two or fifty—will show up and hear the message. They'll hear the call.

Lack of confidence and the need to prove ourselves is about serving our egos. Ever wonder why one person succeeds and we don't? Why are things working out for them and not us? Why do the voices in our heads never, ever stop? I urge you not to worry about this monologue—it's a daily walk and commitment to disregard the mental banter.

I still often find myself seeking ways to quiet my mind. Countless times I sat down to complete this book, and still, weeks, months, years went by and the book didn't get finished.

Why?

For me, it's a drive for perfection. Like I said in the preface, my dang ego wants things perfect before I share them, be they ideas or a manuscript. I put way more thought and energy into what I thought you, the reader, wanted to hear, than I would have by being authentic and revealing what was in my heart.

I understand now that this stems from shunning my internal voice. Not trusting myself. From years of not allowing my own intuitive energy and guides to lead me, but instead, listening to whatever others had to say. I've learned that some of the most prolific artists and successful people have followed their inner guides, allowing themselves not to conform to what others think or say. For instance, Prince, Lady Gaga, Michael Jackson, Versace, and Oprah Winfrey, to name a few.

Alas, I finally did it, and there's the beauty: when you sit down and focus, you can accomplish great things. In a few hours of committed effort, my manuscript grew from 13,200 words to 15,200 words.

Encouraged by my progress, I continued until the book was completed in its raw draft form. After that point, I took a break to relax, quiet my mind, and let the words marinate before I picked it up to read each word.

Finally, I turned it over to an editor to begin the process of dissecting and rewriting.

That progress occurred during the pandemic.

Hair and Accountability

I've already mentioned some of my vulnerabilities, as in my lack of confidence—looking to others for approval and seeking their input on how I should be and what I should do, instead of following my own heart.

But deep down the confidence is there. And I'd bet it's there for most of us.

My blonde hair has always been a confidence booster—a "super power." When I walk into the room and flick my locks, I know I get attention. I'm "the blonde with blue eyes."

I don't mention this out of conceit; it's simply my truth. Many of us have some features we're happy with and those features make us more comfortable with ourselves. We feel more confident because of them. It might be our eye color or long legs, or freckles, or whatever. I know my hair gets positive attention, and I use that to my advantage when I want to feel confident. In many ways I've lacked confidence, or, more accurately, I haven't *felt* confident. However, confidence is locked within us, and for me it's revealed through the power of my hair.

Some people in the world have great confidence around money—making money and being successful. For them, where money comes from is an afterthought.

Other people struggle with money, relationships, or being confident about their looks.

Yet, when we're in the flow of the essence of our being, things will come naturally. And the flow applies to successful relationships, health, money, and looking good. When we're healthy inside, it shows on the outside!

Despite my body image issues with the eating disorder, being attractive has been a core thing since I can remember. Being blue-eyed and blonde, I've been aware of that fact for my entire existence. I've never had a hard time finding a date or being in a relationship.

But I want to be okay with or without hair, with or without a perfect body. I admit my blonde hair is a safety net. I've sought to be comfortable in my own skin, whether I look good or not. I seek to always stand on my own feet and be okay with 1,000 likes or zero likes on my social media posts, 100 friends or 2,500 friends.

Do I know who I am? Do you know who you are?

If I shaved my head tomorrow, would I be okay? Strip identity away and I'd be a plain, simple shell of an exterior me—and my soul. Would I be okay with that? I like to think so. I've worked hard over the years to get there, to fully accept myself simply for being me and nothing more. No blonde hair, no perfect body nor perfect personality—exactly me, whole and full within. Some days I'm okay with who I am, what I'm up to, and what I look and feel like. Other days, I struggle emotionally to exist.

It's okay. I'm beginning to understand this is pretty much normal for us human beings.

Why do I feel like a fraud, a liar, and a cheat as I sit and write this book to inspire others? Because I'm not perfect, I guess. At times I couldn't even help myself, let alone anyone else. I mentioned this earlier and I'm repeating it to remind *myself and you* that being perfect is what our egos and others tell us we must be. Thank goodness, perfection is not what we *have* to be about.

Perfection can be what we individually define it to be, not what others tell us it is.

Like all those who struggle with addictions and disorders, I find my effort to be mindful about choosing food to fuel my body—rather than to fill an emotional void—is a battle I face daily, even now. Not drinking alcohol is a daily choice, too. The moment my mind awakens and my feet hit the floor, I'm scanning my body to see if I can detect the slightest bit of fat or weight loss/gain. *How much does my belly protrude this morning? Am I wearing the pajamas that make me feel fat or thin?*

Oh, wait until I pee, and I can reassess this when my bladder is empty. Then I quickly switch thoughts. *This morning I won't put cream in my coffee. In fact, I'll have tea and fruit to start today off on the right path to losing weight.*

All these thoughts occur in the first thirty seconds of my waking up.

Every. Single. Day.

What happened to waking up and thanking my body? Thanking my heart for beating, my legs for moving, my lungs for breathing? I am alive. I am full of life, and I can hear the rooster crowing, excited for a new day. How about telling myself I'm a glorious being in every way, alive, well, and healthy? Aren't those things to be grateful for?

It's a kinder way to live than what I had chosen to do to myself. And one day, after beginning this book, I woke up and said, "Enough is enough. I'm going to be that nicer person to myself, finally. Living in a prison camp in my head with the constant ridicule is not helping my situation, nor is it being kind to myself or others."

Choosing to eat healthily is an active choice and sometimes not an easy one. I'm always torn between choosing carrots or nonnutritious snacks. It's an almost daily ugly reality. But when I choose to see it from a perspective of kindness, I can choose to align for the greater good of my body and soul. I can see how lucky I am today to have choices.

I'm done spending my energy and time striving for what society deems perfection, wanting to please others, and trying to prove I am worthy and valuable—based on my outer appearance.

Food is my go-to. Since we must eat daily to survive, it's challenging, to say the least, when we use food as our drug of choice. When I quit smoking and eventually quit drinking, I gave up two things plaguing my existence that were emotional crutches.

Of course we don't give up food. Finding a happy balance of living life through its difficulties, moods, and experiences, while eating in a way which promotes good health for body, mind, and spirit can be perceived as hard—if we let it. Food can easily become a pacifier to life. I've learned that food is the fuel serving my body, and over time I've become mindful that the balance is found in what and how I eat.

You can attain that awareness too.

Staying Accountable—It Works

While writing this book I had the biggest breakthrough about choices.

I think about food all day. Some days are easier than others to avoid the pitfalls of overeating. I've learned to dance with my body and have paid attention to the times when those pitfalls seem to be at a higher vibe, like when it's my monthly female cycle. Bloating occurs and I *want* to binge and purge. I must use every bit of mental energy to fight the urges to hop in the car and head to the store and buy boxes of sweet gooey goodies or overeat pizza and any other fatty, greasy foods so I can give myself an excuse to overindulge.

I began 2019 with the commitment to make it the first year I would be abstinent from bingeing and purging. And then we moved into the new farmhouse. It was our first move and major decision. To say it was stressful is an understatement, with my husband and our five dogs, four cats, and a guinea pig. I also had my monthly cycle which includes my battle of the bulge and struggle with bingeing and purging.

I felt out of sorts in various ways. I didn't want to purge in the new house. There is something powerful about a fresh start and I wanted to start things on a clean slate. But, alas, like with any addiction, it takes a fierce commitment to shift old reactions and choose new actions. I failed in my commitment; I binged and purged in the new house.

There were on-and-off encounters with the pink porcelain bowl in the new farm bathroom. But through it all, I kept telling myself I would do better and finally get over the eating disorder.

It was while reading *A Return to Love*, by Marianne Williamson, that I started to dive deeper into finding true love for myself. The book talks about us accepting our bodies the way they are. I also started writing this book, which made me accountable.

Doubts still snuck in.

While my emotional response to the stress and my personal self-doubt was to binge and purge, I knew it wasn't the answer anymore. I ultimately decided that my spirit, my soul, and I mattered more than my addiction did.

Choosing self-destructive ways was no longer an option, so I took the option off the table.

I began to practice. I was abstinent for several months when the urge to binge and purge came back like a tidal wave. I'd increased my workouts and was watching what I ate, but my watching and what I was eating were two totally different things. I was planning the binge, as I often did. I had my sneaky ways to ask my husband when he would be out for the night and for how long. I didn't care what he was doing, but I was planning the purge so I needed to know his itinerary. Remember, my disorder was supposed to be a secret.

I also planned it so he wanted pizza for dinner. Pizza was fun to binge and purge. I pulled out the brownie mix to make brownies so that I had something sweet and cakey to binge on. While the pizza was cooking and I was making salads, I had an epiphany: my cycle was due, *and* I was in the middle of writing this book.

How dare I plan a binge and purge session when I was writing a book to inspire and help others face the demon of this ugly disease of food obsession and eating disorders? I didn't want to face the shame and remorse of the next day. I didn't want to feel crappy after my poor choice. I wanted to fight through it, so while I was cutting the cucumber for the salad, I had the urge *not* to indulge, and changed the course of what I was making.

I still made the pizza for my husband, but I also cooked steamed veggies sprinkled with everything seasoning which is my favorite thing to eat. I put the brownie mix away. I told myself I was not going to binge and purge. I wanted to be accountable to my followers, fans, and supporters. I decided I was going to be accountable to myself and my health. We can start fresh each new d ay.

By making a conscious choice to take a different action despite wanting to binge and purge, I'd chosen a good use of my energy reserves. Even if not giving in to the urge meant occupying my time doing things that had little or no meaning, it was a better use of my energy than bingeing and purging. The action of choosing a different path is where the shift began.

Bingeing and purging results in ugly energy. I made a calculated, deliberate decision to no longer let my life be controlled by food. No more was I willing to let food run—and ruin—my life.

Today I dance to a connected beat with my body. I always ask it how I can best serve it. Not what I *want*, but what's going to serve my body best today in relation to what I choose to eat. Some days I want the cake, some days the orange. I don't resist anymore. I flow with my body. Sometimes I choose to listen to my body, and sometimes I choose what I want.

Whatever I do, I simply flow with it and don't judge it. I don't resist today.

Being kind to our bodies means choosing foods which serve and support our bodies, minds, and souls.

Love the Journey

I've always had a calling on my soul. I've known it since I was a small child, ever since I can remember. It's a knowing that there is something different about me and I need to share that gift with the world.

Can you relate? Perhaps you grew up knowing something was different about you—not in a bad way—but you knew there was a calling on your soul. Maybe you could sing like a bird or play the piano like a pro since you were a little child. Mine was the ability to work with and understand animals. I can read animals, whether it's a dog, cat, snake, horse, or bunny. I'm able to see things about them through their presence.

This isn't a psychic thing; it's a knowing in my spirit and mind about their presence, and it has given me a gift to work with animals my entire career and never get hurt. I have handled many kinds of animals—from alligators and owls, horses and pigs, to rats, cats, and dogs. I followed the path of working with animals right out of high school, getting a job in an animal shelter and later working as an animal control officer during my early twenties.

I knew working with animals was my jam.

But it didn't pay much, so I often lived paycheck to paycheck. I was quickly influenced by others to take another path in my career, like going into sales since it seemed more lucrative. Working with animals, according to others, was not a sustainable vocation.

Due to my low self-esteem and lack of confidence, I followed what others told me, ignoring the things in my heart. I could judge myself harshly for not following my instincts, but truth be told, we all walk our paths, learning along the way. Each job taught me valuable things about life and myself. I don't regret any of the things I have done to earn a living.

So often we're guided by the exterior world, sometimes being told, "No, that's not going to work," or "No, that's not how we do things—the way it works is ...." Those statements assume there is one model and we're supposed to fit into that model to attain the perfect goal. It could be the white picket-fenced house, marriage with kids and a dog or cat, and/or a forty-to-eighty-hour-a-week job making $50,000 a year.

Nope, I never saw myself following the cookie-cutter path.

I admired those who followed their path and blazed the way for others, like Ellen, Oprah, and Lady Gaga. I didn't understand I could do the same until I was in my forties and I turned back to what I have always known—self-awareness of my talent and complete acceptance of, and alignment with, my power and energy.

> When I connected to my true calling, I was able to sit down and follow my heart's calling to create an education farm sanctuary—and then ultimately, write this book.

You have the power to follow your true calling, too.

Sometimes we must walk over many bridges, hop over many pebbles, and slide across a lot of tough stuff to get where we end up. We're always learning, stretching, growing, and building for the next thing. Life is a dance that leads us through many valleys and hills, twisting and turning as we go. Remember, I mentioned earlier you'll need to understand there is a higher power who is on your side?

Often, we're our own biggest obstacle in our quest to fulfill that thing in our hearts. It's taken me forty years, y'all, but I'm okay with that because this journey, although bumpy, has been cool and I've found so much to be grateful for along the way.

When I look back and see the path and the parallels, I get goose bumps. I can clearly see the things I needed to walk through so I could learn the necessary lessons to bring me to this moment.

I love the journey.

Awareness Is Everything

I'm now aware that I tend to commit to something and then doubt the wisdom of my commitment and not stick with it. I get an intuitive hit, like to write this book, and I stall and don't follow through. I get angry when I'm trying to force things to go my way and I get easily frustrated when I'm trying to showcase my abilities.

My internal repetitive dialogue says, *It's too hard,* so I quit and never finish things.

Gads, I almost didn't finish this book!

Being aware of those negative messages is key to breaking their hold over us. When I caught myself saying negative things, I had to adopt a new language and repeat positive mantras over and over: "This is easy, this comes to me easily and effortlessly."

It's far easier to reach for the bag of chips that offers immediate gratification, versus stopping, pausing, and asking my body, *What do you need right now? Is it a glass of water or maybe a handful of blueberries?*

Getting into alignment with my inner being and taking the time to ask what it needs is more powerful and more energy efficient than when I react emotionally.

Reacting causes a snowball effect: When I choose the chips, I eat to fill a void and often overeat, and then hate myself, my body, and my brain for allowing the binge to happen.

Afterward, since I'm no longer purging, I sit there with a gut-wrenching, soul-bruising feeling of disappointment.

It is an ugly spiral, yet there is hope.

Learning from Others

If we don't face our fears and challenges in life, we can't overcome them and chase our dreams. We can follow our hearts by listening to the guidance of our intuitive soul.

That journey is far more important and powerful and worthy of your attention than any other.

Listening to our soul speak the love language of healing and guidance is the real essence of life. It's how we access the joy in life and get to do what we are created to do.

To discover the gift of dancing with the soul and energy that's within and around me, I had to get sober from alcohol and clean of my eating disorder.

And it took a giant leap of faith to trust myself to follow my lifelong passion for animals.

Alcohol and other addictions plague many lives, and I feel lucky to have been able to find recovery and live a new and sober life.

We *all* have a story. Some have the courage to tell it and some don't. Maybe more important, some find the courage to live it and some don't.

Teaching and learning have always been big for me; I love to educate and inspire others and make a difference in the world.

I hope you get inspired one day to tell your story if it's your burning desire to do so. Discussing our experiences with others can be helpful to them and healing for us.

You have something to say, and *someone* needs and wants to hear it. You don't have to write a book. It might be a short story, a post, a blog, or simply inviting someone to tea and sharing your life's lessons with them. Telling your story will help you and the other person. We learn a lot by listening to others.

I sure know I have.

During COVID-19, I observed the CEO of the organization I worked for at the time. She was a strong leader in my life. She was compassionate and articulate.

She chose to address the organization and staff daily during the pandemic, updating us on the organization's stance and where things stood each day. The CEO chose to do those updates live on a workplace platform, allowing anyone in the organization to view and participate. People were encouraged to respond with comments or questions.

While I observed the CEO, I also observed my fellow employees and their responses to the messages. The CEO was gracious and compassionate, and while delivering hard-to-process news, she also encouraged compassion and kindness to be practiced by staff within our own personal communities.

It was inspiring to witness and learn from such a guiding force. As with many organizations and businesses, things were touch-and-go economically, and many organizations were making tough decisions which affected staff and business. For many, it was a sink-or-swim situation.

When the CEO delivered the news that there would be no end-of-year bonuses and no merit increases in 2020, it hit like a punch in the gut. While on one hand I was grateful I still had a job, I also wanted to scream.

My colleagues responded to the delivery of the news with grace and compassion. I did not.

Many were willing to give up the organization's 401-k match if it meant jobs would be saved. I sat in the corner, pouting, angry instead of grateful that I had a job when the rest of the world was crashing and burning. So many people were losing their jobs and having to file for unemployment.

The voices in my head told me:

It's not fair.

Why does this always happen to me?

Why can't I get ahead?

And blah, blah, blah!

Remember when I talked about finding a mentor, someone to be your trusted sounding board? A situation like the one I've sketched for you is a great time to call upon that person for help.

My mentor, friend, and sponsor helped to quiet those voices. She quickly became the voice of reason.

She helped me see the greater picture and release and move the resentful energy through. It was encouraging to understand it was okay to feel the way I felt, as long as I didn't stay there too long.

The recovery process cannot happen unless we feel those emotions and acknowledge them. Get them. Work through them. Move on to better thoughts and actions.

Sitting in the ickiness of the "poor me" syndrome is where we get stuck in self-pity, and I'm telling you honestly, there's nothing positive happening there.

Like the times I focused on one "friend" on Facebook who didn't like, comment, or engage with any of my posts. I easily fixated on that one person and convinced myself it was the end of the world.

I let my thoughts consume me. *One* person won't engage out of a *thousand* friends. I allowed one person to rent all the space in my mind, to consume my thoughts. All I could see was they did not "like" me.

And remember when I recounted of feeling down about my writing after I saw another friend praised for their writing on social media? What I omitted was that I saw someone comment on one of my social media posts, saying they loved what I had written and that I was meant to do the work I am doing, including my writing. They commented that I should write because I'm clever and good at telling stories.

Humans have been trained to gravitate to the negative. We want to focus on the bad stuff being sensationalized by the media. Over time we have been programmed to focus on the bad over the good.

Watch any news station and pay attention to what they report on the most: car crashes, deaths, arrests, political nonsense, and more. I have jokingly said I need to start a news station that focuses on the good happening in the world, but the ratings would be bad and we would get no support since most people want to focus on the gloom and doom. It's what sells and drives ratings.

During the COVID-19 pandemic it was hard not to stay glued to the TV for updates. And I noticed my anxiety escalated during those times. When I was able to step away and breathe in fresh air, I experienced relief from the toxic news anxiety.

And watching that CEO update staff daily in a positive way during a time filled with so much fear and anxiety gave me a fresh perspective.

I grew personally and professionally. Those were life-altering lessons.

Slowing Down to Loosen the Reins

The concept for this book and the title came about after an encounter with a dog on the highway.

April 6, 2019, was a typical weekend morning. I was driving to an AA meeting an hour before the start so I could go for a run first. Tackling two things at one time was my aim.

I loved running to lift my spirits; it was a great way to clear my mind and it was an obsession to stay in shape.

As I drove down the ramp exiting I-95, on my way to park in San Marco, a neighborhood of Jacksonville, Florida, I saw movement off to the side of the road.

I looked closer and could tell it was an animal.

It was 8:00 a.m. on a Sunday, and I was thinking, *What could that possibly be wobbling up the ramp?*

As it raced past my vehicle, I came to a screeching halt.

It was a Jack Russell type of small dog, panting profusely, its tongue hanging out.

I started to back up, but quickly became aware of cars barreling down the ramp towards me. The dog was on the shoulder, headed up the ramp toward the highway.

This little dog had the determination I was too familiar with from my days as an animal control officer. Stray dogs on a mission were not going to be stopped.

I attempted to position my vehicle to get out and call to him, but the dog was focused straight ahead.

So many thoughts raced through my mind.

Someone else will stop, for sure.

I could get on the ramp heading back over the bridge to turn around and come back over and meet this dog on his path—which seemed like the only safe option—but how would I do that and still have time to get my run in?

I need to get this run in.

I can't miss running today.

Why me?

I don't have time for this.

The dog is not going to stop for me, anyway.

Park the car and run back this way and see if you can catch him on foot.

It was like my mind was running its own marathon of thoughts.

I made the decision to go run and ignore the dog. I was so obsessed with my weight and image that I was surely not going to miss a run when I had made up my mind that day to do it.

It was as if missing that one-hour run was going to make the biggest difference in my weight. I was convinced if I didn't run, it was going to be the end of maintaining my body image.

I was obsessed with controlling my weight and at the time had become obsessed with working out. My mind was convinced if I didn't get my run in, it was going to make a huge negative difference in my life.

I could not give up my run that morning, even to try and save a little dog's life.

I caught a glimpse of how rigid I'd become. But that situation was not the only glaring example highlighting my obsession with control.

After running, I attended the AA meeting as planned.

Of course, the meeting ran overtime.

The delay in getting finished triggered another character defect. Meetings that ran over the scheduled hour time frame made me crazy. That morning I stayed long enough to watch people celebrate their milestone anniversaries, but I had my purse on my shoulder and sat on the edge of my seat, ready to bolt out the door.

A man sitting to my left leaned over and I guess he could sense my irritation as I looked at my phone several times to check the time.

The gentleman whispered to me, "Where are you going?"

I knew that *he knew* I wanted to leave in a hurry.

I didn't care. I got up and raced out before the closing prayer. You know, I had things to do! Waiting another five minutes was going to kill my momentum to get things done.

As I sat in my car, I had some realizations.

Why? Why did I always rush through things and life? Why couldn't I loosen up and relax? My husband is so different from me. He always stays for the whole meeting, no matter the amount of extra time. And he often stays even longer to chat with people after the meeting. He wants to know them and let them know him.

I was always in a rush. Someone once told me I was so intense it made *their* skin hurt. I imagined their perception of my intensity was because of my pedal-to-the-metal approach to life.

In that quiet moment of reflection, alone in my car, I heard my internal guide tell me to title the book *Loosen the Reins*.

I was constantly rushing about life, and COVID-19 was causing the whole world to slow down and stop. The incident with Kody the horse made me pause and look at the most important things in life.

Loosen the Reins for the title of this book seemed to fit perfectly.

Whether you're on the ground or in the saddle, the reins on a horse are there to help guide the horse where you want him to go. If you pull up or hold the reins taut, the horse will stop. Sometimes you need a stop, but not if you're planning to move forward. Those tightened reins send the wrong energy to the horse, and your horse will respond with tension and probably not do what you ask.

It's the same way with a dog and a leash. Hold the leash pulled tight and the dog feels the negative energy. He'll respond with fear or anxiety.

I've learned it's the same with life. When I grip so tightly to life with my fists and teeth clenched, while I think I'm in control of the outcome, I'm only prolonging the result I don't want. When I loosen my hold and flow with the energy, life becomes a dance.

Loose reins and a loose leash offer an invitation to play, have fun, be in partnership. Don't we deserve to have a life that includes play, fun, and wholesome partnerships?

The COVID-19 pandemic gave me a free pass to reset the pause button and it showed me I don't need to force things. I learned I can show up for my life in small ways, and make a bigger difference than when I was operating with an iron fist and inflexible attitude.

Being open to learning from others' stories and telling our own are ways we can show up for life.

Turning Fear to Faith

Let's talk about crossing bridges.

Anxiety and fear go hand in hand, and one of my greatest fears is crossing bridges. I know I'm not alone in this arena. Do you avoid bridges?

I once did!

In November of 2018, before I bought the farm, my job at the time sent me and a colleague on a cross-country trip. I was working for an animal rescue organization, and we were transporting a cargo van full of rescue dogs from Texas to Illinois.

It was a lifesaving mission full of heartwarming excitement.

Except I was conscious of the fact that I would be traveling across unfamiliar terrain which could possibly send me over a bridge or two.

There's no sense in sugarcoating it. I was terrified even though I was determined to do what I had promised. Driving through several states while following a mapping system along roadways I was unfamiliar with was scary. Taking a deep breath, I disclosed my fear of bridges with the gal who was copiloting.

What I didn't know—except that I felt more vulnerable than I had since I was a young child in Germany—was that my copilot would help me begin to face a fear I'd had for a very long time.

Having the courage to disclose my phobia was enough to give me the bravery to navigate the unknown high structures in our path.

That kind soul helped me to get braver and more confident. Her patience and understanding were a blessing and, if she reads this, I hope she'll know how important she was to my "bridge" recovery.

My fear of bridges was ingrained from days of drinking and drugging. When under the influence, I had a distorted sense of perception, and panic attacks set in when I couldn't decipher my bearings going over bridges. A fear of heights was likely the root cause of the bridge anxiety.

Having a fear of bridges is ironic for someone living in Jacksonville, Florida, a city with *seven* bridges. It's virtually impossible not to cross a bridge anytime you go north, south, east, or west.

Suspension bridges seemed to give me the most anxiety due to their height and steep incline to reach the top. There's a suspension bridge in Jacksonville—the Dames Point—which I used to avoid, no matter how far out of my way I had to go.

I rerouted when my GPS guided my path toward it, and even pulled over to have another person take the wheel. The bridge raised the most palpable taste of fear in me. Something about the suspension and the incline warped my depth perception. When I rose in elevation, I went into a complete panic.

For a long time, I was able to avoid that bridge. But after I bought the farm, the scary bridge seemed right down the street. It became impossible to avoid without an unreasonable inconvenience. My old antics of avoiding and rerouting now threatened to be a huge disadvantage.

I decided the fear was no longer going to run my life. The first time I went over that bridge, it was in the early hours of the morning as I headed to Orlando on a work trip.

The strangest thing happened when I made the decision to drive over it: I sailed over the bridge like nothing. I got to the bottom on the other side and thought, *Did I just go over that terrifying bridge?*

Yes, I had, and I pep-talked myself on the way back from my trip to go over the same bridge again.

Let's say the rest is history. I've learned that when the light is dim, in the early hours of the morning when the sun is barely up, I don't experience such extreme anxiety. My sense of perception doesn't seem to be as distorted.

It took courage in 2018 to acknowledge my fear out loud to another human being. Her compassion to coach me over bridges along our path enabled me to no longer avoid the one bridge that I feared the most in my hometown.

I'm proud to tell you I have successfully navigated, by myself, all bridges in Jacksonville more times than I can count. I haven't gotten stuck at the top once—my worst visual fear.

Freedom awaits us on the other side of fear. Whether it's a bridge, snakes, or clowns, your fear is only as big as you think it is.

When anxiety or mini panic attacks arise—and they do occasionally—I acknowledge the superficial fear and remind myself I have nothing to worry about. I've navigated the suspension bridge in my hometown numerous times. Today I rarely have any anxiety when I go over any bridge. I've even towed a horse trailer over the big, scary bridge.

That bridge has helped me overcome so many other fears.

What Impression Are You Leaving?

I've learned it's powerful to always be aware of what impression I'm making as I live my life my way. Have you ever been at a store or an event, somewhere public, or maybe in a family situation, when you witnessed someone acting like a completely selfish baby—also known as a jerk—because they didn't get their way?

Maybe they engaged in name-calling, demanded to speak with a manager, or muttered things under their breath while storming around. Maybe they threw things or cursed like a maniac. Their behavior made you cringe, embarrassed for them. Their behavior seemed to come from a place of complete superiority, and they made a scene, being a complete jerk to the cashier or worker of the establishment.

One day I was at the local farm feed store. A woman purchased some hay. The hay was in a trailer outside the store, and to get the hay, a worker had to go out and unload the hay from the trailer.

It was apparent the store was short-staffed.

This customer had a sense she might have to wait a bit and came from a self-entitled place. She gave the cashier attitude and asked rudely, "Someone *is* going to meet me at the trailer, right?"

The person left the store to wait outside, and after a while (I am not sure how long), without anyone from the store coming out to help, the customer stomped back into the store. Despite the other customers in line, she interrupted the cashier to demand that someone unload the hay for her or give her permission to go into the trailer and get it herself.

The self-entitled, impatient uncooperativeness of that customer was ugly and rude. Her inappropriate behavior rippled through the other customers like a negative shockwave.

Have you ever been that person? How many people have witnessed you being a "selfish baby" of a customer?

Yes, I was the immature, impatient, inflexible woman acting like a self-centered, self-entitled, spoiled brat.

The incident has stuck in my mind. I watched the expressions of shock and dismay on the faces of the people waiting for help. I've often wondered how many of those people went home and shared the incident on social media, or told a friend, or recalled that incident when they saw someone else acting like a jerk.

The feelings and the negative vibes I created through my actions surely affected those people. I can remember situations when I witnessed people acting like I did that day—and they stand out in my mind clearly.

I cringe and feel embarrassed for people who act like that. Honestly, such lousy behavior is often caused out of fear. I know I was in fear that day. It was a Saturday, and I was rushing around to get my chores and errands done. I didn't have the time to be at a store so long, but shame on me for going there on a Saturday, when everyone else was shopping.

The manager of the store came out to load the hay for me. Several people had called in sick, which left them short-staffed, and he wasn't going to get lunch that day due to the busyness of the store.

Wow, I felt like I'd put my foot in my mouth. I drove away feeling remorseful. How could I go back to that store?

Like the AA meeting when my impatience bordered on being rude, the feed store blowup was an incident which reinforced my commitment to shifting my energy—to slow down and loosen the reins—because my rude behavior was inappropriate. It wasn't anything I could be proud of. It didn't make the world a better place. And it did nothing for my peace of mind. Peace isn't available to anyone so run by their personal agendas and itineraries that they can't be patient or kind.

We never know what someone else is going through in their personal life at home or at work. On any given day, every human being is trying to get through their day the best way they can. Life is meant to live with joy, even while doing errands. Acting like a fool to people is not the way to act in love. Patience is a form of love and being more patient was what I needed to work on.

We don't change overnight. But through our experiences and lessons, we can shift our energy a notch here and there. We begin, over time, to see the changes reflected in our life.

Choosing kindness for everyone became my motto, and I knew I needed to practice it more. If I ever find the guts to get a tattoo, it will be one that reads #BeKind, right on my wrist, to remind me to be kind to everyone, everything, at every moment, and in every situation.

We're given the opportunity to be grateful and live our life in love and light every moment we're alive. Or we can be enslaved by fear and ego. Today I do my best to choose love and light and do my best not to sweat the small stuff, like having to wait when a store is short-staffed.

I practice looking for grace and ease in all things and extend those gifts to other people.

How a Hat Taught Me a Valuable Lesson

I was out shopping, wearing my #BeKind hat.

Yes, my hat proclaims my innermost spiritual principle, which is to #BeKind. But the encounter I had in the parking lot of the grocery store was anything but being kind.

I encountered a woman in a car blocking the driving aisle as she waited for a parking spot. I had spotted a parking place in the next lane over and wanted to slip into it before anyone else did. Here I was, having to wait for her because she chose to take up the entire driving lane, leaving no room to pass. And no way could I wait two minutes for her to park!

So I didn't. I squeezed by and gave her a nasty look as I passed her.

Obviously, the fact that we'd both be shopping in the same grocery store had slipped right by me. Chances were good we'd even get within speaking distance of one another.

I remembered I was wearing my special hat, and ripped it off. My ugly behavior was nothing that emanated a #BeKind attitude. I had been unfriendly and unkind to the point of being ridiculous. I was embarrassed by my behavior, to say the least.

That was not the only ugly episode I can recall. I'd had a few run-ins on the phone with the city for not picking up our trash, problems with the furniture delivery people, and the people fixing our refrigerator. The series of events were out of my control, resulting in my coming unglued internally, and outwardly taking it out on others.

Oh, and let's not forget when I was working from home, JEA came out and abruptly disconnected our service mid-workday. I got terribly angry. How is anger related to fear? Anything which disrupts our perceived control over our lives is a threat. Feeling like we're in control makes us feel worthy, even superior. It's not a want, it's a need. It's ego-driven. The ego's message says only successful people are in control. Only losers aren't in control of every aspect of their lives. And so our response to the loss of control is usually exceedingly unkind.

Sounds counterproductive, right? It sure is.

Those instances were old behaviors creeping back in after I'd decided to be kinder and more considerate. We grow in our spirit through different levels of awakening and awareness. When I took off my hat outside of the grocery store, I recognized my unkind behavior. And I got to choose a different vibration.

We have the possibility to make a new choice at every given moment! The key is to notice what behaviors and attitudes don't support your best life. If you want to change, you can choose to change.

I've learned that when I surrender and stop trying to control everything, there's a lightness to the way life feels. I'm not in a place of constant angst and struggle. I'm in the flow of life. Going back to my spiritual mantra of Being Kind, when I live with an attitude of kindness in all areas—the way I treat myself and everyone else—the world is a kinder place.

There's a question I've learned in a spiritual program: "Do I want to be right or do I want to be joyful?" I *want* to be joyful. But when being right is more important—the reins tighten and, like my horse tenses up, so does my life.

Being joyful is the answer we need to choose to live in peace, love, and freedom. But choosing to be joyful isn't always our first choice, nor is it the easiest. Our ego and pride will always want us to choose to be right.

So how do I do it? How can you do it? Life can be an easy journey if we let it happen to us and don't resist it. On the other hand, with resistance come challenges and challenges bring about growth. Without growing, would we be able to discover what we can be or do? Humans have ego—pride—so choosing to be joyful must be a conscious choice. There's a 1988 song titled "Don't Worry, Be Happy," by Bobby McFerrin. If you've never heard it, go look it up and listen to it. It's a fun song. A simple song. It's a song I've known for a long time, and it makes more sense to me today than it ever has.

Stop worrying, be happy ... and joyful, a more long-lasting happiness without the ups and downs.

The biggest gift I have to share with the world is that I was a raging bulimic and an alcoholic, and I found a way to pull myself out of the depths of despair. Now I live a life of joy, love, peace, freedom, and complete wholeness. It is a daily walk and a life that transforms every day. And if you've got struggles like mine, I want you to know you can transform your life, too.

We've got egos to deal with in an ego-driven world. We have passions given us by our Creator and the tools to do whatever it is we were made to do. We have strengths, weaknesses, flaws, and gifts.

So the bottom line is that if I can choose peace and joy and making a difference—rather than being controlled by my never-satisfied ego—so can you.

Think about the instances when you had a moment to reflect on your behavior or your attitude. Let those reflections be a learning opportunity. I used to judge myself and condemn myself for my bad or ugly behavior, which in turn fueled more of the same. I've learned not to judge it and to give myself a free pass; I recognize the poor behavior for what it is, while I make a choice, move the energy where I want it, and learn from it.

What impression do you want to leave with people?

What Do We Have to Prove?

As I examined the driving force behind my decisions and actions, I kept coming back to one common thread—I was trying desperately to *prove myself, prove my value, prove I knew more than someone else*, and could do this or that.

I was desperate for approval and to be liked, no matter what the cost. I started to wonder if maybe I wasn't the only one living in such a no-win situation.

How many of us try to prove ourselves or prove something to ourselves?

Social media is a norm. We watch what others post and wonder at the things we read and see. Is there more to what people put on their social media than we get to see? Are they trying to prove themselves? Do we post things to get people to "like" us? Do they post what they do to be "seen" by others?

We've all read self-righteous posts some people put on social media. Maybe they want to be considered an expert in something that they aren't an expert in, except when they're behind a keyboard.

I asked myself if I was doing the same thing. I started to take a long, hard look at my motives. Obviously, what I was doing wasn't working.

It was all or nothing. I wanted everyone to like me. Even the people who could care less about me in any way and made it clear they did not want to be my friend. When we were face-to-face, they said they did, but their actions—or lack of—spoke louder than their words. They never returned my messages, texts, or Facebook likes.

I spent countless hours wondering why one or two people didn't want to be my friend, when hundreds of others did. Why? I had a need to please and be liked by everyone. I found my value in the "likes" of others.

As far back as I can remember, I have always been working at proving myself worthy of friendship, worthy of respect, worthy of a great job, worthy of admiration. I see it behind almost everything I did.

Like road rage. Which is all about the ego.

As soon as *How dare you!* comes screaming into our minds, our ego has us by the throat. Road rage is posturing: to prove our car is bigger, more expensive, or faster. We *should* be first or we are a better driver than the person we cut off—or who cut us off, right?

Why is there such a need to prove our value and worth? Why do we "kill" ourselves day in and day out, packing our schedules to the max to get more done, to say we've accomplished the impossible? More doesn't equal better.

It's as if everyone and everything is an obstacle for us to get around and get past so we can go on to the next thing. These are times when we're not viewing people through the eyes of God—we're viewing people through the eyes of competition. That competition is our ego encouraging us to think we must prove ourselves better than everyone else at everything. When ego is running the show, our guard is always up in defense to what we perceive others are thinking about us. *We feel like they are always judging us, and in turn we are always judging others.*

> For forty plus years I've been working at letting go of the need to prove myself; I'm a work in progress. I reach different levels of surrender in each situation I encounter.

I'm constantly hoping for our rescue horses to demonstrate that they like me. If they pull away from me, I interpret their reaction to mean they don't love me, so therefore I'm unworthy of love. That response is like how I felt about the one individual who didn't like me or ignored me on social media.

I take this "proving stuff" to prayer a lot and ask why I care so much about who likes me or not. I also ask for direction regarding what to do with the nonprofit work and what I should be focused on.

The message is often: *When you accept that you are already whole and complete inside, you won't care about what individual people think or say. When you feel worthy of accepting my gifts, I (God) will give you the moon.*

How do I feel worthy? How do I feel worthy from the inside out? I asked.

Validate yourself in me. Know that you are valuable and lovable because I love you.

Let's face it, we're born with an intuitive guide—every person has intuition. Whether we want to listen and trust it is up to us. Some of us are more in tune with it and some of us suppress our inner guidance due to experiences we've encountered in our lives. I blocked my intuitive guide years ago and began to rediscover it within the last several years.

As I've said earlier, I've always sensed or felt a calling on my heart and soul—one I was aware of early in life. That calling was crystal clear and it came up often—but anytime I followed it, I suppressed it. People told me this passion would never amount to anything and that I needed to find a "real" career path—something which would pay the bills, since working with animals wasn't going to get me anywhere fast.

The suppression of my intuitive guide created a power struggle within me that left my ego in charge. So I was always out to prove myself, which led to feelings of unworthiness. Finding my way back to tuning in and listening to my own inner guide was the greatest thing I ever did.

Forgiveness

I've had to do a lot of forgiving to reach a place of complete surrender. Getting sober required a lot of forgiveness. I love to tell this story; it's part of my past and a powerful illustration of complete forgiveness.

I was living in New England when my drinking and eating disorders were full-blown. I went to a local bar down the street, within walking distance of where I lived. My friends hung out there and it was convenient for a drunk like me: no risk of a DUI and I was bound to be safe while I drank myself into oblivion.

One time, the bartender—who was only doing her job—recognized I'd had too much to drink and refused to serve me. This drunk girl didn't like it and I proceeded to make a scene. I called her vulgar names that would appall anyone with a sense of decency. I was immediately banned from the establishment.

Banishment was devastating for this alcoholic and I didn't know what I was going to do.

So I did what any selfish human being would do; I found a way to get back into that bar to drink with my friends. I wrote a letter of apology and asked for a second chance to be able to visit the bar with my friends again. Kind of like offering amends, only my request for forgiveness was purely selfish. I wanted to be able to drink in the bar with everyone else.

I didn't care about the poor bartender's feelings, nor my own dignity and respect. I didn't care I'd embarrassed my friends. I look back and think what a sad state of existence I was in then.

Through my recovery process, I've learned to forgive myself for those awful events. They were driven by alcohol, and I wasn't thinking like a kind and caring human being with a heart for life and others. That isn't an excuse, mind you, but it is a way to understand who I was at the time.

Today I have forgiveness for myself. I spend much less time judging myself. Instead, I can analyze any actions, reactions, and attitudes that don't support my life's mantra of #BeKind, and adjust.

I'm not perfect and I've done imperfect things I was once ashamed of. I can look upon them and know they shaped my life's course. They influenced who I am today and the message I share with the world. While I don't condone my past behavior, I do see it in a new light and I don't judge it. It's okay. In the same way I have forgiveness for others, I have forgiveness for myself—a ton of forgiveness. Today I give myself the grace to be a work in progress.

The Disease to Please

You can't put me in a box. I like chocolate, but I'm particular about what I like. Yes, I like the flavor, but only for certain things. I *do not* like chocolate cake, no matter how you make it. Layer it with fluffy white icing, and I'll eat the icing off the top and leave the cake behind.

I love dark chocolate, but I'm not a big fan of milk chocolate. I dislike anything that's double chocolate, unless, of course, it's a Tootsie Pop, and my favorite flavor is—you guessed it—the chocolate, which is chocolate on chocolate.

I know this chocolate thing about myself is a part of my unique blueprint. I wouldn't alter or change this chocolate thing about me, yet I'd contort myself to fit in a box on other things simply because I wanted to be liked.

People play games and ask silly questions on social media all the time. One game was to list ten things "I" (meaning the person playing and posting the answers) don't like that "most" everyone else loves or at least likes. I don't normally play those games, but that one caught my attention and I engaged. Two things immediately came to mind:

1. Pasta

2. Jeans

Pasta, how could I not love pasta?

I will tell you why in another chapter, so for now let's focus on the jeans.

Jeans are a human fashion staple, it seems. "Jeans are pants made from denim or dungaree cloth. They were invented by Jacob Davis and Levi Strauss in 1873 and are worn still, but in a different context. Jeans are named after the city of Genoa in Italy, a place where cotton corduroy, called either jean or jeane, was manufactured." (www.thehistoryofjeans.com, 2020.)

Millions of people wear jeans today, from the mines to the boardroom. Dressed up or dressed down, jeans are versatile and evolving in the fashion world. They are worn around the globe. But I was never a fan; I loathe jeans.

Jeans have never been flattering to my figure. The only reason why I have worn them is because I felt pressured to wear them, pressured to believe that jeans were the cool thing to wear. In my perspective, jeans make me look fat. A crazy thought, right? Not to someone looking for approval from everyone but herself. And certainly not to someone with an image disorder.

That influence of what others thought I should do versus what called to my heart and soul is a part of the backbone to this book. As a people pleaser, I've always done what others thought I should or shouldn't do. It seems, until my mid-forties, my entire existence was the result of what others thought I should do, and not what Jessie wanted or thought was best for her or the situation. I didn't know how to think for myself.

I call it the "disease to please," and I sacrificed my own health and grounding to put more emphasis on how everyone around me felt or would feel if I chose to do X or Y. The disease to please ultimately cost me every single time.

Give me khakis or leggings over jeans any day. As a horse enthusiast and as I ventured into the horse world, I slowly realized jeans were a cowboy and cowgirl thing. But as a forty-year-old starting out with my horse passion, I was more grounded in my own awareness of who I was and honestly didn't get into the jean-wearing thing.

I chose to make my own fashion rules, wearing muck boots with shorts, spandex leggings, and workout gear instead. It has been an exercise in learning to be okay in my own skin and to follow my own sense of comfort and fashion.

The horses and animals at the farm sanctuary have helped me find my voice and faith in myself. I've learned that being kind to myself means allowing myself to be authentically *me*.

A Way to Exhale and Heal

My lack of trust in myself and others has shown up in many forms. When working with horses you can't force anything. You can't be rushed. Working with them takes time. The vibe of force (my way or no way) and ego (they will do as I want) has shown its ugly head as I work with these horses and other farm animals. I've tried to force their acceptance and friendship and it doesn't work with them—or with anyone, actually.

Imagine going on a first date with someone and, within the first hour of sitting down to dinner, asking them to get married and have kids. Any sane person would head for the door and fast! And, trust me, I've done that with men during my dating years. I still remember bringing up the conversation of marriage during those heavy drinking days. Clearly, I wasn't thinking straight.

The topic of kids wasn't relevant to me. Having children was not part of my story and I've known that since I was young. The poor guys who got subjected to my heavy cross-examination right away—please forgive me if you read this. I certainly had a lot of internal growing up to do.

I've lacked trust in myself, and I've discovered it goes back to the lack of healing surrounding the loss of my friend. Food filled the void for many years. Food was a comforting thing and something I could control and make friends with right away. Today I'm learning that horses and others play an integral role in our healing. In addition, writing has given me healing and solace. I highly recommend it if you're working through stuff of your own.

Finding a notebook or journal to write in is a great start. What many find cathartic about writing is that we can safely release what we keep inside. We will never hurt the feeling of a journal or piece of paper. The things I bottled up or buried deep inside got released and flowed onto a piece of paper. Getting stuff out and onto paper helps to move the energy around it.

Find a journal that resonates with you. It might have a pretty pattern on it or have a hard cover with a spiral or clasp closure. Look around and choose the one which not only catches your eye but gets you excited to own it. A special journal is more fun to pick up and write in, so choose a journal with a design that speaks to your soul. Begin writing in it. And you may find that if you journal during a time when you are reading a good book, you'll tap into the energy that is invoked by the ideas and subjects discussed. It's empowering to the soul.

Many books contributed to my healing. I'd always journal about the things that stoked a spark in my soul. If something I was reading caused a riff or invoked a deeper sense of searching within me, I'd write it down and explore it when I had time. I loved to write things down and journal about them.

Often, I have reread books and discovered something new. Many books have a lot of concepts in their pages to process, and we may be at different levels of our spiritual learning each time we read them. When rereading books, we find new things that resonate with us.

This chapter has been healing for me; I have reopened some of my journals and I can see the levels of healing I've been through. I can see where I played the tape repeatedly, year after year. And I can see how far I've come in my spiritual growth since my lost days of alcohol and food abuse.

Many times, I prayed to God and I used my journals to write to God, as if writing a letter to my father or best friend. I asked for relief and asked God to allow me to be okay with my body: let me be okay with how it looked or felt, no matter what.

I wanted desperately to be okay with my outer shell and stop living in the prison of my brain. It's crazy to see how many times I prayed and wrote for relief. Often, I felt relief because writing is such a tool for release. Repetition gets more stuff out, constantly and consistently. It certainly does not need to be divulged to anyone el se.

You don't have to lay bare your inner journal writing with the world, but putting pen to paper relieves the pressure of holding it in. Try it. If you're afraid someone will read it, get a few pieces of paper and write freely. You can burn or shred the papers when you're done. This isn't about chronicling your life; it's about release—letting things go that bind you up emotionally and spiritually. It's not about recording your pain, but more about releasing whatever bothers you. Get it out of your captive soul. Send it into the sunlight of the spirit.

Let stuff go and trust the process of release. Find a quiet place to sit. Start writing and don't stop until you feel relief. You may have to write a few times to get it out and to keep letting it go when you find stuff creeps back up. That's normal for this process. We became trapped by old stuff and negative messages over time, so it makes sense that it will take some time to peel back those layers, get them out, and let them go.

This book isn't the first time I've written about Sarah or my eating disorder. I've done a ton of writing over the years. I have many journals about the stuff surrounding the loss of my friend and the struggles of bingeing and purging, but the writing is where the magic happens.

Every time I write, I get a little lighter. Each release brings forth more freedom for my heart and soul. My pain around the issues I write about has become more joyful and the memories become fonder. I celebrate Sarah's life more now and I'm grateful for the friendship I had with her.

Let your journal be the vehicle in which healing takes place.

Writing in a journal is not rocket science. Many people have written books on the endeavor of journaling, so of course it's not my idea. When we read or hear the same things time after time, seeds for healing get planted again and again. Eventually, for our own good, we need to step forth and make a change. Writing things out, reading them, and writing them again are ways we can make ourselves light enough to take the leap.

When will you make that change happen for yourself?

Writing is an outlet. I release whatever is rolling around in my head. When we hold on to something bothersome and stuff it down into our subconscious, that's when we get into trouble. We're not dealing with what is going on emotionally. We shift to food and other things to soothe a wound or avoid the healing which needs to occur.

I wanted to continue to call Sarah and write her letters, like I had done before her accident. Eagerly awaiting her mailed responses was so much fun as a child, like having a pen pal whom I knew and loved. I wanted to grow old and see where our lives would lead and lean on each other for support as we navigated life as teenagers, adults, building families together and apart. I missed out on that, and I desperately craved it from the moment she left the planet.

I was overwhelmed with hopelessness when I couldn't say goodbye. I coped with my grief through lies. I convinced myself that people—especially friends—don't matter that much. Nothing and no one should be a big deal, so the pain wouldn't be devastating.

Building new friendships was hard; I was afraid everyone was going to leave me. I understand now where that belief comes from, and I no longer bury it or discard my feelings as if they don't matter.

Today I acknowledge my feelings and I'm able to do it because I write and release the emotions constructively. Writing has also helped me to build trust in myself. When I write, I can see and feel the emotions and it builds confidence and trust.

I've also learned to trust myself through experiences with the animals.

Sharing to Live on Purpose Today

Remember the CEO who helped me by being an inspiring leader? Well, while I was having my pity party about no bonus or pay increase, the CEO offered a severance package to the employees. That's not common in the nonprofit sector.

A companywide offer to leave with a severance? That CEO did it. She wanted people working for the organization who were invested in the mission.

I was not. While I loved the work they were doing for animals in our nation, I was committed to a deeper cause of kindness and compassion through EPIC Outreach. I thought long and hard, evaluated the pros and cons, looked within, and listened to the guidance of my heart. I saw the severance as a clear sign. It was time to move forward.

I took the severance offer, a leap of faith that I was going to find a way to make the mission of EPIC Outreach and my writing, my purpose.

Each time I prayed, asking God to reveal the direction I should go with my life, I was directed to share my story. I always thought I needed some grandiose idea to make my life have meaning or purpose. But I was shown that I have a story to tell: the story of overcoming a more than twenty-year battle with an eating disorder. Many people struggle with bulimia daily and cannot see a way out. I found a way to be free, and now I'm so grateful, I'm going to broadcast it to the world.

While alcohol caused chaos in my life—and it was not how I wanted to live—the eating disorder is what had me in a vise grip.

It ran my life and influenced my drinking. I drank to erase the ugliness the eating disorder created within me. I hated myself and saw myself as someone who never looked as good as everyone else, so I forfeited 99.9 percent of my self-esteem for an unattainable and unsustainable outer image.

When I stopped bingeing and purging, it was the epicentral act of being kind to myself. And when COVID-19 happened, I had to slow down, take a step back, and evaluate my life. The things I'd been studying—slowing down, less is more, slow is faster—started coming together, and I began to look within and evaluate how I was treating myself. I began to respond and act differently to myself, my life, and those around me as I started to understand that our answers lie within.

Moving forward, I'm constantly evolving. We never "arrive" in life, we keep peeling the onion back, building the salad one ingredient at a time, and opening ourselves more to the learning of who we are and what we're doing or are meant to be doing. We and our "mission" change over time. And that's okay. I don't have to have it all figured out right now, and neither do you.

The little stories and experiences I've mentioned have led me to where I am today, living my life on purpose, with kindness at the center. That's what it's about. When I reread some of the stories in this book, I see them as learning opportunities. It's strange to read them; I can see how much I've grown—and it's like, wow, did I once live like that and act like that and do those ugly things?

I did. I can own my mistakes, fears, and immaturity without judgment. I can forgive myself and keep working every day to be a stronger, more joyful person on a mission to do good in the world. To grow hope for those who need it. To heal and encourage where I can. That's life—always evolving, always changing. We grow with the ebbs and flows of it. One day I'll write another book to pass along the things I've learned since publishing *this* book. I already have the new book started in my mind.

Today I live on purpose, and a dear friend taught me how.

Live Like Laura

Living on purpose is so much easier and more powerful. Buying a farm and having a horse is my purpose and my truth. Choose your life and don't worry about being perfect or getting it perfect. To achieve my power and courage, I had to let go of perfection. I'd been plagued with bulimia for so long, due to my obsession with perfection. It's something I've had to learn and still remind myself of every day. And when I experience little snippets of my purpose, it reinforces the importance of that very thing: to live on *purpose*!

Meet my friend Laura. She had a grace about her, an ease with life. She was young, beautiful, and full of life. She exuded what everyone wants to be and have. She was liked by so many, and it wasn't a challenge for her to be liked by many. It came naturally to her and for her.

Sadly, sweet Laura passed away in a tragic car accident at a young age. There's a theme surrounding her memory: #LiveLikeLaura. To me, that embodies living carefree and full of life. She was a breath of fresh air. She had vitality for life.

I think about her often and attempt to live my life like her.

She loved a particular Scripture from the Bible, Romans 12:2: "Do not conform to the pattern of this world but be transformed by the renewing of your mind. Then you will be able to test and approve what God's will is—his good, pleasing, and perfect will." It is so in line with the thread of how I live my life today. Changing how I think changes how I act and how I live on purpose.

I've learned to celebrate life and not worry so much about what others think of me. I say, celebrate those who support you and forget the rest. If your side of the street is clean, the issues aren't about you, they're about them. I can't control whatever someone else is dealing with in their life; I can only control myself and my issues. I don't worry about winning every "like" or "follow." I've discovered I've already wasted far too much time worrying about what was wrong with me because someone didn't like me. That was not living like Laura.

Today, life ebbs and flows. It's 2024 and my manuscript is now a published book. I've been sober from drugs and alcohol for fifteen years and abstinent from bulimia for five years. Each passing year is better and better.

While this memoir is a record of my journey to a new life of being kind to myself, there is still more evolving to do. Staying abstinent from any vice—unhealthy food, alcohol, drugs—is something I work on daily. It's a spiritual walk, so it doesn't feel like work. The following pages will reveal more of what life is like today: how I arrived at these moments and how they're leading to more awareness and growth for my soul.

Raising My Consciousness

I started tuning in to the great works of Esther Hicks, who channels a collective spirit named Abraham, and they have transformed my journey of self-love to another level. Esther is a spiritual thought leader I was introduced to while discovering a new raised consciousness. I fell in love with Esther's teachings. They helped me to dig deep, tapping into my subconscious mind. I took it upon myself to discover her more by researching her and absorbing as much as I could.

I Googled "weight loss and Abraham Hicks" and "Abraham Hicks and attracting abundance" and "Abraham Hicks and self-worth." You'll find many videos of her teachings at YouTube, for anyone's viewing, and they're eight to fifteen minutes long (some shorter or longer). I watched as many as I could, and more than once.

I've learned to allow things to soak in and set in. As they take root in my spirit, a change begins to occur. It's like building a muscle. You build it over time. Change can happen quickly if you let it, but it does take persistence and commitment. I'm still evolving by listening to Abraham and Esther's great teachings, along with teachings from Wayne Dyer, Louise Hay, and Bob Proctor.

Abraham-Hicks has a common instruction: "Be tuned in, tapped in, turned on," which means to be in alignment with how I feel. To listen to how I feel and check in with what I'm doing or thinking or feeling; to be conscious or aware of myself and my emotions and thoughts. It's a daily walk, like staying sober from drugs and alcohol.

One of the tools I've applied—apart from listening and studying great thought leaders—is EFT tapping. EFT stands for Emotional Freedom Techniques. This technique stimulates the twelve meridian acupressure points of the body to relieve symptoms of a negative experience or emotion. I'm not an expert on the hows and whys of EFT, so please take some time to research it for yourself.

Tapping has helped me reshape the thoughts, ideas, and actions of who I am and what I'm doing. I have taken the time to study tapping and have even worked with someone one-on-one to learn the technique. Applying this technique has helped me approach things more calmly and it changes the wave patterns in my consciousness. Tapping changes the tempo of our internal vibrations.

Tapping has been helpful with changing how I respond to what I eat. I have always bought carrots and celery with the best intentions, and I do like carrots and celery, but they're not my first choice of foods. If there are crackers or pretzels, peanuts, or granola, I'll choose those salty snacks instead. Always!

I like to eat healthy things not just for my waistline, but for my heart. Choosing healthier foods when they are readily available in the fridge takes practice and a conscious choice. It's like rearranging the neurons in the wave pattern in my brain. It's like getting sober and choosing a new way of life. Through consistent repeated behavior, we create new patterns.

Tapping helps that.

It's like changing our words to create a new reality. When we tell ourselves "That house is ugly," then of course it's ugly. If we tell ourselves we're sick or fat or we're coming down with an illness or a cold, of course we are—it's what we believe.

What You Believe, You Will Receive

Change your vocabulary and you will see a different result. See things differently and the world will change right before your eyes, literally.

For example, I read a friend's post on social media lamenting rental properties being so expensive. They were complaining about never being able to get out on their own since rents were so high and landlords wanted deposits and so on. At the time, they were in their forties and still living at home with their parents. The post on social media was negative and the finger was pointed at everyone else being the cause of the problem.

We create our own reality and if we're living in poverty, it's due to our poverty mindset, plain and simple.

In a fundraising social media group, I saw someone share a goal to raise $950,000 to buy a property that would provide shelter for the animals the woman was rescuing. She was running the rescue out of her home and it was not working. The need to help quickly outgrew her capacity to help.

The woman's post received a great deal of "logical" feedback encouraging her to start small. Some of the responses were from long-standing organizations coaching her to be patient because it could take her twenty years or more to raise that kind of money. The larger organizations explained they had a larger donor base which had taken them some time to create, build, and nurture.

The person who posted that grandiose vision and goal was so disappointed with the comments that she left the group. I reached out to her privately and encouraged her. I told her if she believed in energy work and trusted that raising the $950,000 was part of her calling, she should get out and do it.

We can't let anything stop us. Once we get into alignment with the thing we're supposed to be doing, it will happen like magic and probably won't require twenty years to create. It can manifest overnight. Man is limited by time frames, not by our Creator.

Everything we touch is a stepping stone to our inner growth journey. Everything we do leads us to more awakening in our soul, heart, and mind.

Sharing a Breakthrough to Inspire You

Here is a personal story of how manifesting happens when we are aligned with the thing we're supposed to be doing.

On February 5, 2020, I was practicing energy work and trusting the process of growing my nonprofit, EPIC Outreach. I made a commitment to work at getting the nonprofit to be self-sustaining in 2020, without relying on my personal financial support. I also had the vision to see it surpass operational fundraising support so I could leave my day job by the end of 2020 and work the nonprofit full-time, year-round, being fully supported by the work.

A part of the nonprofit's mission is rescuing animals that are a great fit for humane education outreach. Now, I've told you I worry about what others think of me, and that carries over to second-guessing myself in the work I do. I had, in the past, worried about what others thought about the decisions I made with the nonprofit.

As I stepped into a new paradigm of doing things differently, I challenged myself that week in February and took a risk in posting on social media about a new horse we were planning to take in. I worked with my tapping coach at the time to dial into the guidance of why we were taking the horse in. I wasn't doing it for a personal reason; this horse needed a sanctuary home and was a perfect fit for our nonprofit's mission.

> It was a challenge to post about the horse on social media; I wasn't sure what the response would be. I was terrified of failure. I was hoping for a positive response, but worried about a negative backlash and no support.

To my surprise, that post on Facebook received nearly one hundred likes, with multiple comments. At the time, that was considered a lot of engagement. I remember thinking, *Why do I doubt myself? When I'm in alignment with my true path, everything lines up and people are supportive.*

I posted a Facebook fundraiser which I had been shying away from because, yes, I hated the idea that it could fail. If I post a fundraiser and it doesn't reach the goal—which is rare—I assign the poor performance as a personal failure, as though I'm the one who isn't worthy of people's support.

But I was taking steps toward building my trust muscle. I created the fundraiser with the mindset that regardless of the results, I was taking an action step with this nonprofit. Fundraising is what I do. And more important, I wholeheartedly believe in the work and mission of the nonprofit. Seeking support from the community is the only way to sustain it and continue to make a difference.

I invited my friends to the fundraiser on Facebook, and in less than twenty-four hours the fundraiser had almost reached the goal of $1,000. People who didn't typically donate came through. I was blown away by the response, and again questioned why I had doubted myself and the purpose of EPIC.

In the field of manifestations, this is considered the work of building trust. Building trust is a process. And I was on my way to trusting myself, trusting what I was out to create in the universe, and working at telling doubt to take a hike—it isn't allowed in my creative energy.

You can do this, too.

For forty plus years my life felt like a merry-go-round; it seemed like it kept going around and around, always coming back to the same desperate place. Sometimes I felt a little wiser and a little further along in my personal growth, but I still had a deep longing for something more. I was never satisfied with anything. I got the job, the farm, the horses ... but I needed donkeys, and maybe a pony. I wanted more, more, more.

Nothing, and I mean nothing, was enough.

I was eight months into living on the farm when I started hearing the message to slow down and loosen the reins: stop trying to prove myself. The horses played a big part in that. Horses are spiritual creatures, and they don't tolerate being manhandled or treated badly. They respond to spirit and energy, and when there is good energy, the response is great.

I noticed magic happens when you connect after spending time with them. The connection also includes grooming them, letting them nuzzle and smell you as you sit on a bench in their space. That's worth more than riding the horse—simply spending time with them.

For the longest time I thought if I had horses, I must ride them.

No.

My spending time on the ground, caring for them and loving them and being with them, is where it happens. Showing them my love is what I do.

In October of 2019 I started to implement what my heart and spirit were suggesting. Prior to that I was living a suffocating life. I woke up in paradise, living my life's dream, but I was suffocating from the drive to be perfect and striving to figure it out myself. I forgot that I could stop trying to do everything on my own and I could call upon my spirit for guidance.

Nuggets I Have Learned from Abraham-Hicks

The teachings of Abraham through Esther Hicks have transformed my life. She has reshaped how I see things, think about things, and how I respond and navigate life. She talks about how the universe and all things, including humans, are a vibration. And life happens based on vibrations, thoughts, and feelings.

"A vibration becomes a thought, and a thought becomes reality from the feelings." The better it feels, the more you are leaning in the direction of where you want to go. Nothing exists in your desires that you cannot bring into existence.

You must believe you are a receiver. Stop thinking it is about *action*—it's not. You are a vibrational being in a vibrational universe. There is a vibrational existence that exists in fullness, and we must tune in to access it. We need to care about how we feel because it's about feelings. Everything in the universe is a vibration.

- Conscious, deliberate thought

- Focused – be focused

- All good things come

- Vibrational beings in a vibrational universe

- Live on purpose

When we gain control of our vibration, we gain control of how we feel. Then we don't live in constant *reaction* to our circumstances and current conditions. We can't want the condition to be the way we want it to be for us to feel good.

It will never work that way.

For example: If you want a husband in order to be joyful, or require money in the bank before you'll be joyful, you'll have a big problem.

You must be joyful *first*, and then the right husband and money will show up.

The thought and the emotion (feeling) must be there before the result shows up. Sometimes it takes time to fully manifest. If I need the full manifested version to show up before I feel good, I won't feel good for a while. Maybe never. Find the feeling of it—focus to keep the feeling and it will manifest fast. Feel good about what you don't have—yet.

I realize this is a difficult concept to grasp. Our world is a "show me" world. We've become skeptics of our own power, which keeps us powerless! Feel the vibrational essence of what you want and the reality of it will appear quickly. In biblical terms, this is what the apostle, Paul, wrote about from prison, when he told followers: "In every circumstance, I have learned to be content." Being in alignment with our purpose is how contentment is experienced and learned.

I stopped worrying about the things I didn't have, and I started to identify what I felt in my spirit about why I wanted them. As I focused on the feeling, it's as if I already had it, and before I could turn around, there it was.

Learning from YouTube

As I mentioned, Abraham-Hicks has a lot of YouTube videos that are free to watch.

In one of the fifteen-minute videos, Abraham discusses finding peace with food, and this is what Esther shared that turned things around for me:

"Make peace with your food and never get fat."

She talked about coming into alignment with who we are and what we're doing. Most often, people scarf their food down and are never present to why or what they eat. We are too worried about what we're going to eat, how it's going to affect our body, how much should we eat, when should we eat, and the concerns go on.

Many of you, right now, are probably thinking about food in some form or fashion and when you're going to eat next, or perhaps you are eating while you read this book. Abraham asked how many of us knew people who "ate like horses" and never got fat. We watch them eat all kinds of stuff and wonder how they could eat like that—whether it be cakes and cookies or fried food or breads and pastries—and stay so thin.

Haven't we also heard people announce, "I can eat anything I want and never get fat."

Huh? What? How is that possible?

Here's why. They *know* they can eat whatever they want and they'll never get fat. They don't think about metabolism and how many calories something has, they eat whatever they want in any quantity and they never get fat. Why? They are in alignment with the concept that they can eat whatever they want and never get fat.

Abraham went on to explain that if you and I talk to our bodies, show love to ourselves, and get into alignment and agreement, our bodies and every cell within it will do what it knows to do with the food we put into our bodies. We're to listen to our bodies and spirit. When we're in alignment, anything we choose to eat, in any quantity, we can eat and not get fat. When we're in alignment we will follow the guidance of our body, mind, and spirit and will choose the foods which serve our bodies best.

I know this seems like a lot to "digest" about Abraham-Hicks, but I encourage you to explore Abraham-Hicks.com and read or view the teachings via the web. They cover many subjects.

It could transform your life like it did mine.

Break off from reading this and go infuse your mind and soul. I want you to discover a thought leader for yourself, as I did. If not Esther Hicks, find another leader who resonates with you and learn the power of positivity from them.

Small Talk about Horses

During a time when I was working as a recruiter for a nonprofit organization, I interviewed people all day long, day after day, week after week. I loved the job because I got to speak with many people across the country. We each have stories to tell, and people from all occupations have gone places to do cool things.

Building relationships as I got acquainted with the candidates was fun and opened my mind to new things. I often went down "bunny trails" when people mentioned anything to do with horses. I was working that job during my early days of learning about horse care. In one interview, the interviewee and I talked about how intuitive horses are.

It was during the time I was challenged with communicating with the horse named Kody. I wasn't connected with him. I'd watch him and sense he was troubled and scared. After chatting with the interviewee, I decided to spend a little extra time with Kody that afternoon. We worked together with the halter on, and afterwards I gave him space to come up to me on his terms.

I waited and waited and waited.

I watched him. I could feel he distrusted me ... fearful of what might happen if we got close. After giving him more time, I could see the wheels turn and it was as if a sigh of relief came over him. His whole body relaxed, and he walked right up to me because *he* wanted to. Or was it because I wanted him to? Hmm ....

It was incredibly amazing.

Teddy the Mule: Less Is More, Slow Is Faster

I was blessed to have had the farm sanctuary during the COVID-19 pandemic. The farm allowed me to step away from the stresses of a world gone mad and get that mental and physical relief we all needed. Stepping away meant I spent more time with the animals. And more time with them was where I learned the lesson, "Less is more, slow is faster."

Teddy the mule taught me the power of slowing down. The farm sanctuary rescued Teddy in the summer of 2020, in the middle of the pandemic, from a local animal control agency. EPIC Outreach was asked to help, and I went out on a limb trusting I would be shown how to help him when I knew nothing about mules.

I wanted to help and I wanted to learn.

Teddy had been found running loose. Imagine a large brown mule walking freely down the road. I imagine it was a sight to see. Teddy was untrusting to the point I couldn't even get a halter and lead on him.

I was fortunate to have met an experienced mule rescue partner from Texas who became a tremendous help. She guided me and inspired me virtually. She taught me that slow is faster and less is more when working with mules. She advised me to not push his trust. Over a few weeks of using the method of going slow and doing less, I was able to place the halter on him.

It was like the stars aligned and the sun sparkled for us that day.

It was so rewarding to earn his trust. And one day, I was standing in the sand after I had gotten him on the halter and lead, and I moved to touch a foot as if I was going to lift it off the ground. I had no intention of doing anything except begin the process of earning his trust by lifting a foot for a hoof trim. To my surprise, he instantly lifted his front foot as if we had practiced him lifting it for me a million times.

It was so automatic it was insane.

After the shock wore off, I stood there and instantly started crying tears of "Holy shitake, he trusted me and gave me his foot!"

I was proud I'd trusted myself enough to keep going and working with him, when on so any levels I'd wanted to give up and ask someone else to take him. I'm so glad I didn't give up.

I learned a lot from Teddy about trust.

And a lot about less is more and slow is faster.

I am the harshest judge of myself, and I put many barriers and limitations on myself. The horses reflect that back to me. How I approach them dictates their response. When I'm rushed and controlling, they're not so giving and easy to work with. When I'm slow and gentle, things work like a dance with them.

While COVID-19 brought the world—in a weird way—to a time of healing, I'm unraveling one buckle, one harness, one halter at a time when I work with the horses and spend time at a slower pace on the farm.

At the farm I can use my unique experiences, which include learning through hands-on encounters with large, intelligent, and highly intuitive beings. I've learned I must slow down to communicate with them. When I let my ego get in the way—and it sometimes does—I must either step back from the animal engagement or not engage at all.

I've learned to step back and pray, meditate, tap and recenter myself, or take a break.

When I'm trying to assert myself or I let ego take over, I'll get kicked at or the animal won't have anything to do with me. Now, that's what I'd call an ego deflater!

Many times, I'll walk out to the barn to work with the animals and I'm aware my ego is a little flared. Anxiety is sitting in my chest. I'm rushing to get things done and I feel overwhelmed by the mountain of things on my to-do list. In those moments, I can choose to stand in the pasture with the donkeys and be still until the anxiety subsides. That puts the ego to rest—I have nothing to prove to anyone. I can be present to the animals who are ego-free beings. Having the animals near often brings on a sense of calm.

The power of noticing we're out of alignment is that we can fix it, and fast. I ask my body and spirit what's going on. What do I need to be aware of? I can also ask the universe what the goal for the training or encounter is and realign myself to nonjudgment or no expectations for the outcome.

I can let the animals direct the outcome through what they want or will allow. In other words, I leave it up to them. Through these interactions I have begun to redefine who I am as a person. As I continue to develop, refine, and grow in my soul development, I am learning as much as I can from the animals; they will always be my greatest teachers.

Kindness and compassion can't exist if ego is present—unless you let ego serve you by being an uplifting energy to move you forward and spark a desire for change for the betterment of all.

Ego: do you serve it or do you let it serve you?

Ego will always exist; it's part of being human. How we respond to our ego is where we have a choice. What are we choosing today?

Our egos play a huge part in our relationship with our physical bodies, our relationships with animals and people, and with the world as a whole.

More Lessons from the Horses

Buddy is an older horse we took on as a project. He was an exceptionally large horse and pure white—reminding me of a unicorn. He was used as a camp horse for kids and had recently retired to living on a farm with other horses. He was being pushed around and not getting the food he needed to maintain his weight. He was underweight and needed a new path. We decided to take him in since his demeanor was perfect for working with kids in our education outreach.

After caring for him for several months, it was obvious he wasn't gaining enough weight. I was awakening myself to the energy of *my* body and food. I couldn't figure out why I couldn't help this horse; I worked hard not to consider it all my failure in some way.

Since I was learning to ask myself what my body and spirit needed daily, I thought perhaps I could do the same thing with Buddy. I went and spent some one-on-one time with Buddy and asked him intuitively what he needed. What did his body call for and what did he ultimately want and need? The energy message I received was that Buddy needed a rescuer who knew how to help him.

> I was not the right rescuer; I was still learning about horses and their care. I was too new at horse rehabilitation to know how to help Buddy and I knew in my spirit what I had to do.

While I did my best for Buddy at the time, he needed a place which specialized in skinny horses. So, while some might judge letting a horse go to another rescue facility as a failure, I, for the first time, saw it as a stepping stone.

Buddy came to EPIC Outreach as part of his path to get the best overall care for his future. Another rescue organization I had a relationship with took Buddy and rehabbed him to perfect health. Buddy returned to EPIC Outreach about a year later, and all we had to do was maintain his weight. He has done a phenomenal job as an ambassador to kids and adults, and he has fully sustained his weight long-term.

I believe that when we dance with energy, we will always be guided to the right path and right action for the highest good of all. Buddy is a perfect example of how I live my life today, tuning in to the energy and asking intuitive questions, seeking guidance from within.

Energy Work

Energy, to me, is using the vibration that moves through my body and the cells that make up my outer shell. It's the sun warming my bones, heating my body when I sit and let it soak in.

I've found that when I tune in to my body and connect to the energy within, I'm able to appreciate my body and let my inner guide tell me what is best for my physical and spiritual needs. I appreciate every part of my body, thanking it for taking care of me and protecting me all these years.

Our bodies know how to care for us in the best way.

I learned a great acronym in Alcoholics Anonymous. HALT: Hungry, Angry, Lonely, Tired. We learn that any time those negative tapes start playing and the old ego kicks up the anxiety levels, we need to use HALT to find out what has triggered us. Have we eaten? Are we angry about something and, if so, what? Are we lonely and do we need to reach out to our sponsor or another trusted support person? Have we gotten enough rest?

While that originally helped me get sober, I also use the HALT concept to keep my body healthy. I have applied this tool to the eating disorder. When I find I'm challenged by something in my life that throws me off course and I seek food for comfort, before I indulge in a bag of pretzels I pause and look to see if I am Hungry, Angry, Lonely, or Tired.

It's like shifting the perspective on things.

I started loving my body. Part of my prayer and meditation routine was a time I called "loving me." I scanned my body, head to toe, and was thankful for every inch, every toe, every cell, all my organs, all my muscles, and I thanked them for being healthy and carrying me this far in life, and for providing a healthy vessel to carry me for 112 years. (I have claimed that age for a long time and believe with every fiber of my being that I will live to be that age.)

You might find that HALT can help you to take better care of yourself, too!

Things I Did and Do

Here is what I did:

- I surrounded myself with things that encouraged me, guided me, and empowered me. I listened to inspirational thought leaders online.

- I made a commitment and stuck to it. I wanted it more than life. It was a life-or-death decision. I either got better or I died. Period.

Things I Did and Do, That You Can Do to Redirect the Bingeing and Purging, or Anything That You Find Is Occupying Your Focus, Like Alcohol, Drugs, Overspending, and So On

- **Make the decision that you are going to stop.** I made the decision to *stop*! I made it definite and never looked back. Bingeing and purging was no longer an option. I stopped giving myself permission to give in to the urges and self-will desires.

I stopped drinking and drugging.

I stopped bingeing and purging.

I stopped doing what others thought I "should" do, and followed my heart and inner guidance. I made the decision to write this book.

Making the decision was when I actually was able to stop drinking, bingeing, purging, and I set my mind to writing this book. I stopped saying "Someday" or "I will start on Monday," or "I will change when I have more time, a new job, when things are different," and the list goes on.

You must feel the conviction: *I am committed to making a shift and to stop doing the thing I am conditioned to do.*

Whatever has your focus is likely a habit by now.

The only way to stop is to have the conviction of your decision and stop. And then begin to take new actions toward your new vision.

In 2009 I made a clear decision to quit drinking; in 2019 I stopped bingeing and purging; in 2022 I made the decision to finish writing this book and publish it. Once I'd made my decision, I declared my commitment to the decision, followed guided direction, and took action to support the decision.

I went to Alcoholics Anonymous meetings, I worked a 12-step program for the alcohol and bulimia, and I scheduled the time to write. I wouldn't let anything get in the way of going to meetings with AA, and recently I kept my commitment to writing by letting others know I had a commitment to a personal project.

On my calendar, I scheduled time to write. I never quit. I got it done.

Once we make the decision to stop or change or make something positive happen, it becomes a turning point. Then we must seek knowledge from those who are qualified to teach us, listen to the messages, follow our intuitive guide, and constantly seek more awakening.

There will still be things to overcome along the way, but the biggest hurdle is making the decision.

In 2023 I saw a pattern when I kept avoiding writing. I found every excuse to do other things other than write this memoir. I kept telling myself I'd complete it someday, and I would see bios of people my age who had completed multiple books already. The only difference between them and me is that they got it done.

When I realized I was avoiding the calling on my soul to complete this book, I buckled down.

Once I made the decision and commitment to get this book done, things began to flow. I got visions of what this book would and could be and how it would touch the lives of many people in so many ways. I began to feel the contents. New visions, new stories, and fresh ideas began rolling in. It was phenomenal.

Within forty-eight hours, I birthed a new book in its purest form and in the best light and love possible—I literally co-created with the universe. It was amazing!

- **Learn to trust.** Building trust in all areas of my life has been where I've grown the most. I've learned to trust the process in everything.

I have a mantra that everything is working out for my greatest good. Trust is layered. Building my trust muscle has come through working with the rescued animals, and every day I feel like it gets strengthened through various experiences.

I also learned to trust by listening to and watching other people.

My husband is the type of guy who is influential. If someone tells him to do something and he trusts them, he does what they say. I'm more skeptical.

A spiritual guide friend of mine reminds me that I often say, "Things work out for you, but not for me." That statement aligns me with the energy of things not working out because I've had an old belief system of skepticism.

One day I was praying and laughing at how my husband had done an energetic treatment with a device which uses energy waves to stimulate circulation in your cells and blood. At the time, he was having pain in his hip and other joints. I'd received the same treatment from the energy wave, and I, of course, didn't feel anything from the treatment. Since there was no difference in the way I felt, I decided the treatment didn't work.

Well, my husband, after receiving only two treatments, exclaimed, "I feel better today! It must be the energy device." He believed it would work and trusted it was working. The aha was that I realized since he believed it would work, it did, and he felt better.

What? In all my energy work, I know that many of the things we experience are based on our belief system and what we have programmed our subconscious mind to believe. Trusting something to work is enough, and consistently believing something works retrains our subconscious to believe.

In that moment I "got it," and the aha reinforced the fact that I could trust the process of manifesting my own beliefs. Now, would I manifest positive outcomes or negative ones?

- **Learn to let go.** It's a daily practice of letting go and realigning to my authentic self.

Every day I ask myself what my body needs to be nurtured and fulfilled.

Some days are better than others. Some days I say yes to the cupcake, some days I listen and drink the water.

Every day the voices in my head guide me one way while my spirit says to go another way. But it's when I slow down and do the thing my inner being guides me to do—that's where the magic is. It's a daily practice of connecting with yoga, prayer, meditation, writing, and connecting with others (accountability).

I do this to stay sober.

Getting sober saved my life. Without sobriety, I have no idea where I would be, so I say never look at your hurdles as wrongs. They may be the very things that save your life.

Getting sober was the catalyst for my becoming abstinent from my eating disorder. It's the daily walk of redefining who I am every day, month to month, and year to year that defines who I am. But to get there, it took letting go of my old patterns of living.

I often say to myself: *I choose my body, I choose me. I love my body, I love me. The more I love my body, the more money comes to me.*

I share this chant because little mantras help me get through the times when I'm being hard on myself or walking through old triggers, such as comparing myself to others. They might help you, as well. When I look at past pictures of myself and see the body image I loved and sometimes crave, I remind myself that the old pictures are from a time when I was bingeing and purging, and I don't want that body if it comes at the price of self-destructive behaviors. It might look nearly perfect, but inside I was living a dying disease, chained by a negative and destructive internal argument. I resisted what my body craved to be and forced myself to be and look like someone society told me was better.

Appearances aren't everything. What you see on the outside ... remember, you have no idea what's happening on the inside. Letting go and changing my perception to accept who I am and what my body wants and needs to be, gets easier the more I practice it.

Encouraging each other to love ourselves the way we are is the most beautiful thing we can do.

Lifting each other up is choosing to be kinder to ourselves and each other, but it doesn't change the internal mental and physical struggle we still face living in our own bodies, sometimes feeling captive.

Again, I give myself more grace today than I ever have before; I'm less likely to beat myself up. Rather, I embrace the glory that my body is—strength, endurance, lifesaving, and inspiring.

- **Get a buddy.** An accountability partner.

Having a mentor is paramount to anyone's success.

Surrounding ourselves with things that encourage us, guide us, and empower us is critical to being successful in changing. Support might be an in-person buddy or two, or inspirational thought leaders you can access online.

In the program of Alcoholics Anonymous we have sponsors, so I have a sponsor who points out the things I cannot see for myself. I check in with my sponsor daily and we talk weekly about what's going on in my life.

A buddy or accountability partner will help you see things you can't see for yourself. They're a lifesaver and even when you think you're probably exhausting them, unless they *tell you* you're exhausting them, keep seeking and asking for guidance.

We need people to help us walk through life. Life is an ongoing work in progress. If you haven't found the right accountability partner, keep looking until you do.

You need someone who won't sugarcoat things and will have the endurance to repeat the same message until you get it. And let's face it, sometimes it takes repetition because we bump into various situations that are triggers.

Unraveling our learned automatic responses to triggers takes time. But we *can* undo old patterns and create new patterns for living.

Each time we think we've finally gotten something, it seems we're faced with a new circumstance and need to unravel a bit more. So, having someone to walk with you through life's circumstances and point out the things we keep getting tripped up on is *huge*—really *huge*—due to the fact we can't see those things for ourselves.

A buddy will help you get to a place of self-acceptance.

It's like planting a seed. Each planted seed, when thoughtfully cared for, eventually grows and blossoms. The more seeds you plant, the more will grow and blossom.

I was a vegetarian at the age of fifteen. I never liked meat and only ate it when I had to. When we ate burgers from the grill, I wanted a cheeseburger and usually ate the cheese and the bun and left the burger. When I was asked to eat steak or meatloaf, I would drown it in ketchup—I disliked the taste. But I loved cheese.

I ate cheese but no eggs, milk, or any animal meat. I understood cheese was made from milk, but I think subconsciously I blocked it and, then again, didn't realize that cows, goats, and sheep are exploited for their milk and all its byproducts. I still felt it was safe and humane to eat.

Vegan people here and there told me about where cheese came from. I read things and heard things. It never sunk in. I started to explore plant-based cheeses. Since I couldn't find one I liked, I wasn't committed to making the shift.

One day I met a friend for smoothies, to talk about life and catch up. Somehow, we began to talk about the subject of veganism. She asked me about eating cheese, and another seed was planted about consuming cheese.

I'm not sure why. Or how. But that day the conversation sunk in.

It wasn't her genius way of explaining things; she didn't say anything I hadn't already heard. Her intention wasn't to make me change my mind. She was simply sharing information.

But all those other seeds, along with hers, sprouted. I made it a priority to find a plant-based cheese that I liked and stop eating dairy cheese. Since that day, I rarely eat any kind of cheese unless it's plant-based cheese. There is only plant-based cheese in my fridge. The only time I might eat real cheese is when I'm out and forget to ask someone to hold the cheese or if there are no alternatives.

Having a buddy, an accountability partner, someone to deliver the same message over and over until it sinks in will help you shift in your own life.

It works and it makes all the difference. It's what has helped me stay abstinent from bingeing and purging.

- **Know your triggers.** Another way I stay abstinent is through an understanding of what my trigger foods are.

I know what types of things will send me into a mental tailspin. I know my trigger foods.

Remember my mention of pasta a few chapters back?

Pasta dates to Marco Polo; it is believed that he introduced pasta from China, but according to The History of Pasta at wannapasta.com, "noodles in Italy date back to times of the Etruscans and the Romans. Recipes including pasta can be traced back as far as 800 A.D., some believing it could have been as long ago as 1 A.D." Almost every country has a version of pasta—it's such a widely known and loved dish. It's an ideal carbohydrate that can be light and airy and mixed with so many different foods, from cool summer dishes to warm dinner entrées.

To me, pasta was fun and easy to inhale in so many different forms, and it was one of those easy foods to binge and purge.

Pasta is one of my trigger foods. I am aware of how it makes me feel, so I avoid it.

People are amazed that I do not eat pasta—like jaw-dropping amazed. Who doesn't love pasta? I love it, but it isn't good for me.

My inner guide, my mantra, my past experiences tell me to stay the heck away from pasta; it doesn't serve my soul or my emotions positively in any way.

Bagels, those chewy things we slather with cream cheese, butter, or jelly? My taste buds water at the mention of an everything bagel. Salt, poppy seeds, garlic: they overload my senses.

I love bagels, but I don't eat them. They are a trigger.

The same is true for brownies, those ooey-gooey chocolatey things that melt in our mouths, especially if covered with chocolate icing.

Bagels and brownies are trigger foods: if I eat them, I'm triggered to want to binge and purge. They are the indulgent foods that sink to the bottom of my stomach like a rock and call to my brain, yelling, *"You're going to get fat, you'd better get rid of that food."*

And every time I eat those rich foods and move my body any which way, I am reminded at every turn that I have indulged in "bad" foods and that's the reason I'm fat, even though I'm not fat.

Whenever I ate those foods, among others like crackers, cookies, and cakes, I overindulged until I couldn't eat any more and then I had to purge.

So, these and other types of foods trigger those old negative messages and my ego insists I must hate myself. I have learned to not judge myself for eating or looking at certain foods and making them wrong or bad. And while I never want to resist or deny myself any type of food, I do know what foods aren't good choices if I want to stay grounded in compassion and kindness for myself.

- **I do not weigh myself.** Trigger foods are not the only things which send me into a tailspin; so does weighing myself.

How many of you have a scale at home? Perhaps you weigh yourself at the gym.

When I go to the doctor and they want to update my weight and ask me to get on the scale, I am not too prideful to ask them not to say the number out loud. Even if it's only one or two pounds over what I think I weigh.

Weight as a number is enough to send me down the rabbit hole of obsessing.

These days, I'm not willing to play on that court.

Instead, I judge my weight gain on how my clothes fit and how I feel about myself. I know every inch of my being and I can tell if I have gained weight or not.

I don't need a scale to tell me the news.

I've learned to ask my body what it needs to serve the cells within. If I listen, it will always tell me. It's up to me to listen and follow the guidance.

I've also stopped comparing. I am not perfect at the no-comparing thing, but I do my best to catch when I'm in comparison mode. I've begun to practice looking for ways we're alike, instead of different.

And I've surrendered to not having a perfect body.

What is a perfect body, anyway?

Is it what I reference in a magazine or a commercial? Or is it the thing I tap into when I ask my soul, *What size and shape do you want to be?*

Do I let my body dictate what it looks like, or do I let my ego, which imposes an unrealistic image of what shape is best for my body?

My body knows best, not my ego.

My motto these days: "My body chooses what shape it wants to be."

If I listen to the guidance and follow its lead, I will always be perfect despite my shape or size. And my shape or size may ebb and flow with the seasons, depending on the food options or fitness levels at any given time.

And it's okay and everything is perfect the way it is at any specific moment.

Choose One Step That Resonates with You and Implement It Today

Shifting our beliefs or actions takes time. I've mentioned the actions that have worked for me and for many others, yet there is always room for growth.

Right before the printing of this memoir I found myself in a massive funk. I was struggling with some compassion fatigue. The subject of compassion fatigue is its own topic. What I came to be aware of is that my body and how I feel in my body significantly influence how I feel physically and emotionally.

I quickly realized I'd been eating emotionally, a lot!

The amount of pressure I was under running the farm sanctuary, fundraising, and rescuing animals was super heavy and weighing on me emotionally.

All of the social media, animal care, emails, phone calls, managing volunteers, events, and rescue requests—at the time felt overwhelming.

I had to take a long look and say *Stop!*

I was emotionally eating to fill a void, using food to nourish and replenish my soul. Was I hungry? No. Was I angry? No. Was I lonely? Nope. Was I tired? You bet!

I was also aligning to the thing I labeled as "compassion fatigue."

I had a heated argument with my husband (I call arguments moments of moving energy, and it's healthy to have arguments) that had me look long and deep at what was going on in my spirit. I took a few minutes and sat quietly asking my spirit guides for help.

I heard the message: *Stop aligning to the things you don't want. You keep attracting them.*

I was not only *feeling* compassion fatigue, but I was *telling* people I was dealing with it. Energetically, I kept aligning with compassion fatigue.

I was feeling like a victim of this fatigue. I was, in a sense, resisting my own well-being.

I've learned through studying thought leaders that we are energetic beings and we're naturally well in our mind, body, and spirit. But we have to align ourselves to the wellness that is always available.

As I sat in the quiet, God, my higher power, said, *"You may feel this way now and you may have had an argument a few minutes ago with your husband, but you can shift how you feel right now."*

We can shift the course of the next few minutes, hours, and day by changing how we feel and how we react moving forward. We can change the course and path of our immediate future.

> The past doesn't have to dictate the future—shift it right now by choosing differently.

I did!

For the next thirty days, I shifted to noticing how I felt and how I responded to the life I was living. I stopped emotionally eating, and whenever I recognized I was using food to fill a void, I stopped and changed my behavior.

I saw dramatic results not only physically, but in my emotional state, in my energy level, and in my self-esteem.

I was no longer a victim of my ego and my emotions; I was in charge of creating my future life of joy and purpose.

A Note of Encouragement

Have you ever had a nagging urge to do something, but you couldn't make yourself do it?

Since I've become a published author with a few children's books, people often tell me they have a book lodged in their brain that they haven't had the courage to write. They mention they don't know how to do it and they want to know how I made it happen.

I can relate to their fears because writing this book—sitting down to collect my thoughts and experiences into a condensed "manual" to share with the world—has been one of my greatest challenges. I have never been able to figure out exactly why, but what I can say is the demons have been a huge hurdle and facing them down has been a huge blessing. Facing the biggest demon of our lives is not easy.

From the moment my eyes opened in the morning to when they closed at night, I used to struggle with eating. I wondered daily if the struggle would ever end. Today my brain and my body live in synergy, but I must stay vigilant and in the positive mindset I've worked so hard to make mine.

If you have a battle going on in your head, I promise there is relief. I'm a girl who has dealt with the battle of eating—and drinking—for more years than I like to admit. I've been able to turn the tables, literally, and make a difference for myself, and you can do it, too.

At some time, we get to a point where enough is enough. We make the decision.

It was around March or April of 2019 when I said "Enough!" It was like, *Am I going to keep wasting my energy bingeing and purging or spend time with the animals on the farm?* Spending time in the bathroom had lost its appeal and its hold over me.

Remember: change takes time. It involves layers of work within. I had to pray, meditate, work, and engage with others. I had to build a network of trusted sponsors and supporters to help me stay truthful and strong. I had to surrender my addictions and insecurities to God, my higher power. Over time—after years of self-development—I'm in a place where I can write my books and blossom. We each have our own path of self-discovery. And it starts with giving yourself permission to make that declaration and get on the road to change!

I haven't arrived; there is still more to discover and uncover.

However, I'm not where I was yesterday. At this moment I may not be entirely where I want to be, but I'm on my way. For some people it may take less time to see a transformational change and for some it may take longer. None of that matters.

Don't be discouraged; it's reality, and we have to give ourselves permission to fall down and not beat ourselves up. We get back up, brush ourselves off, and start again. No judgments. No self-loathing. Goodness knows, I self-crucified all the time—there is no space for that today! Today there's only space for love and kindness for me and all who cross my path.

Step aside from the torment.

Rewriting My Contract with the Universe

When I eat, I'm trusting food for my comfort—when I should be trusting God, the universe, a higher being than me. Rewriting my contract with the universe means I have to rewrite how I speak and think and how I respond to life. Most of the time my reaction is based on feelings and listening to my ego. It took me a long time to learn to respond by listening to a higher power which guides and directs me.

Like everyone else, I must make decisions every day; I'm either going to follow a path of least resistance, which means to listen to my soul guidance, or I am going to fight and do it my way, which will be the harder way. I have noticed when I choose the harder way, it's because I either don't want to do what is being asked of me or I don't like what I hear.

Making the decision to choose a spiritual path isn't an easy one. When I discussed journaling a few chapters back, you'll remember I mentioned that writing things out is about taking a different approach and seeking a different result. If what we have done in the past wasn't working to bring us peace, joy, and love for ourselves, in life, and for others, isn't it time to change things up? I knew I kept showing up empty-handed, yet continued doing the same things anyway.

In summary, most of my life I've put way too much stock into what others thought was a better way for me. I chose alternate jobs because people said I couldn't make money working with animals. I chose to binge and purge because the world said only skinny women were wanted and desirable. I didn't do things, thinking I needed to know about every relevant aspect before I could be, do, or have those things.

I'm learning that we can all do, be, or have anything we want to do, be, or have. Starting is probably the hardest part. We can learn as we go.

One Action, EPIC Impact

It's always been my intention to inspire the world, to help the planet be a more compassionate place for all living things. I have a dream to pass along information, be a public speaker and educator, and to encourage others to be kinder to each other, themselves, the planet, and animals. I have a dream to urge kids to be kinder to themselves and each other through their learning to be empathetic to animals and the planet. When kids are compassionate and kind to each other, we'll have created a more compassionate and kinder community and world. Interaction with our EPIC animals allows children to learn empathy, patience, and gentleness.

I've given talks on this subject: One Action, EPIC Impact.

All anyone has to do is take one action. Maybe it's sharing something positive on social media or calling a friend to say hello—one action to make a difference. COVID-19 was a prime example of how small actions make big differences. We saw people step up and make masks to give co-workers; people shopped for their neighbors; and families did a drive-by visit to wish loved ones a happy birthday during the times of social distancing. Kindness does not need to be heroic or extraordinary; we're everyday people getting into action to make a difference for someone else.

Everything is possible if we loosen the reins and slow down to notice and enjoy life.

Lacking resources is not the problem; lacking resourcefulness is.

Change your story, you'll change your life.

Why Did I Write This Book?

Why is this book in your hands?

I'm no one special, most would say. I don't have a talk show, I'm not rich and famous (yet, but I am on my way), and I'm not a social media sensation (yet). However, I am someone with a passion to encourage. Why shouldn't I tell my story? The same goes for you. You are somebody with something to say that will help someone else. Why tether ourselves to an internal conversation that says we don't have anything worthwhile to contribute to others? That is possibly the biggest lie of all!

The topics of bulimia, eating disorders, and addictions of any kind are not the topics of choice for many. It's uncomfortable for people to discuss. But unless we give ourselves the grace to talk about uncomfortable topics, people will continue to suffer and succumb to things that can be overcome. There are people who care and will help on the road to recovery, but they can't help if they don't know what the challenge is.

I want to inspire people to follow their path. I want to encourage people to get to know themselves and treat themselves with love and respect and kindness. When we follow what calls to our hearts, we're in alignment with the greatest thing that could ever be.

Wayne Dyer says, "Don't die with your music still in you." That quote has stayed with me since I heard him say it. I don't want to get to the end of my life and wish I had told my story or followed my heart and done what I had thought about day and night. Nope, I want to do it all, and say, "Wow, that was a really great ride." And I want the same for you.

I hope by writing this book I help someone else become and stay abstinent from an eating disorder or any ailment or addiction plaguing them.

This book is my way to open the door to allow healing to take place. The calling to inspire people—to raise their consciousness to make better decisions for themselves, others, animals, and the planet—is something I've had for a long time. Sometimes my calling may seem overwhelming and pointless; however, this book is a vehicle, a message of permission so others can tell themselves, "Hey, stop striving for perfection."

When we strive for perfection, we let ego get in our way. It prevents us from doing the next right thing. We want to always shine, we want to always be right, and never raise our hand to admit we are wrong or that we need help.

Look at politics from this perspective. Ego drives the decisions. If politics was driven by doing the next right thing for all, and decisions were made for the best interest of others and not driven by money or gaining votes, things would be drastically different in the world.

I want you to see my vulnerability. I want you to understand I'm nobody special in the grand scheme of things, but I *am* willing to be an example. I have raised my hand and said, "I need help. I don't know how to do this."

That was and is sometimes hard to do. I don't like to admit I don't know what I'm doing or that I need help, but I've learned it's the only way to improve at something.

Asking for help is not a weakness or an imperfection, it's a strength. Humility is a strength. Kindness is a strength. Relying on others loosens the reins on life and allows others to step up, step in, and step out to help us.

While I hope one day I get to meet you in person, meeting you virtually via the words on these pages is spectacular, too. Believe me when I say I can't wait to meet you! Relationships never used to be important to me, but today they are everything. They're the building blocks to so many great things.

I put getting healthy and sound-minded at the front of the Great Things list. I say "getting" because I'm still evolving—still learning. As you know, my transformation didn't happen overnight; I made decisions which stopped my downward spirals and led to this new life that brings me a great deal of joy and peace. It took lots of internal work and still takes a commitment to grow spiritually and mentally and to stay abstinent and sober.

You, too, can heal and grow. Whatever the mind can conceive and believe, it can achieve.

Remember to be kind to yourself. Loosen the reins on your life, and I promise all things are possible.

My Hope for You

Today I slow things down by listening to intuitive and creative guidance. I might take a walk in the pasture in my bare feet, participate in a coaching program, or get quiet through meditation. I turn everything over to my higher power, ask for guidance and alignment for what I want to create, and follow my intuition.

And whether I'm sitting in the hammock surrounded by the animals I have rescued—who might be rustling around beneath me—or when I engage them in play or training, they are my greatest teachers. They light my fire. My story is about the things I learn from spending time with the animals. That's the leap of faith I've taken, to follow my God-given talents so I can live my authentic life.

As a work in progress, I have opportunities to practice everything I've told you. And if I can do it, so can you. We're not alone in this life—we do it together.

This is a little prayer I've said to myself and prayed many times: "You are a child of God. He is supplying all your needs and desires. Abundant prosperous wealth is on its way and here to stay. God, I surrender EPIC Outreach to you. You know my heart and you gave me this passion. It's not where I want or thought it would be. I leave it in your hands. I trust you. I trust you. I trust and believe. I know and I receive. I trust you as I put pen to paper. I trust that the right decision is being made clear to me today. I trust that all things with the farm are working out for all good."

Do you have a nudge? It doesn't have to be to write a book. It can be anything. Maybe it's to volunteer or get involved in something more aligned to your heart's calling. Maybe it's to sail around the world or start a baking business. Whatever your nudge is, I beg you, don't ignore it. If there is one thing I can inspire or encourage you to do, it's to follow the nudge within you that's calling to your heart—even if at first you doubt you can achieve it.

I didn't know anything about horses until I started volunteering, and a year after that I bought a seven-acre farm, took in my first two horses, and the rest is history.

Get started on following your heart. You only live once, and ignoring the nudge is like denying your soul the whole purpose of its existence.

It's with deepest gratitude and love that I wish you all the best in your quest for freedom in your life. Nothing in life is sweeter than being freed from the things holding us back. I hope this book has inspired you to step up, step out, and step into the life you have been called to, and that you will start following the dream within—and not look back.

Find your dream, find your path, and go after it. Find the alignment within. You know what that is for you. Whatever has been nagging at your heart and soul—go do it! Stop making excuses and go after it.

If a behavior, addiction, or eating disorder is holding you back, stop making excuses and do something about it. Remember, you don't overcome these things overnight, yet as soon as you make the decision to do something about it, the faster it will unravel and you will overcome it. I promise.

Whatever your heart's desire, loosen the reins, slow down, hit the pause button. Enjoy the person you are today. We can and need to do this on a regular basis. It's what we all need to live our best life. And I believe it's what our planet needs most of all.

Be Kind to yourself! And live a life that brings you joy and peace. You deserve it. You are worth it. You are magnificent!

Organizations

To learn more about the organizations mentioned in this book, please visit:

Alcoholics Anonymous – https://www.AA.org

Overeaters Anonymous – https://www/OA.org

EPIC Outreach – https://www.EpicOutreach.org

About the Author

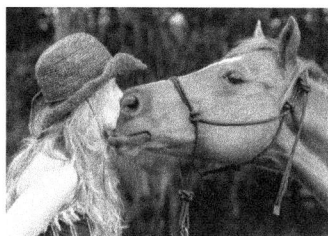

Author Jessie Miller is an animal activist whose journey to make a difference in the world began when she was young. At the impressionable age of ten, she witnessed a tragic incident involving a German shepherd that had been hit by a car. The sight of the motionless and helpless dog sparked a deep sense of compassion. She questioned why nobody took action and why no one seemed to care. At that moment Jessie knew she had a greater calling in her life.

Over the years Jessie has dedicated herself to animal rescue and outreach, using her experiences in various corporate roles to shape her personality and drive to make a difference for animals, people, and the planet. In 2015, divine inspiration led her to establish EPIC Outreach, an organization with a mission to inspire compassion and create a kinder world for all.

At the heart of EPIC Outreach's work is the belief that compassion can be taught, and Jessie has been instrumental in spreading this message for over thirty years. Through rescue efforts, networking, and educational outreach, she has positively touched the lives of countless animals and people.

In 2019, Jessie's dedication to creating a kinder world led to the expansion of EPIC Outreach, with the creation of a sanctuary where rescued farm animals find a safe haven and serve as education ambassadors. This farm has become a place where children and adults alike can strengthen their human-animal connection and learn about compassion firsthand. This is also where Jessie had an encounter with a horse named Kody—which changed the path of her eating addiction and helped her become abstinent from bulimia.

As an author, Jessie is committed to spreading the message of compassion through various channels. Whether it's children's books, educational outreach programs, or in-person and virtual tours of the sanctuary, Jessie and EPIC Outreach continue to inspire and teach compassion to individuals of all ages.

Jessie's road to peace and making a difference is a testament to the life-changing power of compassion and the profound consequence a single encounter can have on one's life. From her early days of witnessing suffering on the streets to establishing a sanctuary that educates and uplifts, she has overcome personal obstacles, including an eating disorder and alcohol addiction, using her passion for animals and the planet as a driving force.

Through her work with EPIC Outreach, Jessie invites others to join her in creating a kinder world for people, animals, and the planet. Her story serves as a beacon of hope, showing that with dedication and a leap of faith, every individual has the power to make a difference.

Also by Jessie Miller

Other titles by or with Jessie Miller can be found at Amazon.com and through the website www.EpicOutreach.org.

Winnie: A Wet and Windy Adventure

Chance: Wings of Hope

Wrigley: The Wonder Dog

Farm Tales Series with Stephanie Itle-Clark

Oliver's Big Problem

Flock of Friends

Brave Cat, Barn Cat

www.ingramcontent.com/pod-product-compliance
Lightning Source LLC
Chambersburg PA
CBHW070839300326
41935CB00038B/1146